WMC

PRACTICAL OPHTHALMOLOGY

Commissioning Editor: Michael Parkinson
Project Development Manager: Hannah Kenner
Project Manager: Nancy Arnott
Design Direction: George Ajayi
Illustration Manager: Bruce Hogarth
Illustrators: Jane Fallow and Antbits

PRACTICAL OPHTHALMOLOGY
A SURVIVAL GUIDE FOR DOCTORS AND OPTOMETRISTS

Anthony Pane MBBS (Hons) MMedSc FRANZCO
Consultant Ophthalmic Surgeon
Mater Hospital
Brisbane, Australia

Peter Simcock MB ChB DO FRCS MRCP FRCOphth
Consultant Ophthalmic Surgeon
West of England Eye Unit
Royal Devon and Exeter Hospital
Exeter, UK

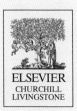

ELSEVIER
CHURCHILL
LIVINGSTONE

Edinburgh London New York Oxford Philadelphia St Louis Sydney Toronto 2005

ELSEVIER
CHURCHILL
LIVINGSTONE

First published 2005
ISBN 0-0443-10112-4

British Library Cataloguing in Publication Data
A catalogue record for this book is available from the British Library

Library of Congress Cataloging in Publication Data
A catalog record for this book is available from the Library of Congress

Notice
Medical knowledge is constantly changing. Standard safety precautions must be followed, but as new research and clinical experience broaden our knowledge, changes in treatment and drug therapy may become necessary or appropriate. Readers are advised to check the most current product information provided by the manufacturer of each drug to be administered to verify the recommended dose, the method and duration of administration, and contraindications. It is the responsibility of the practitioner, relying on experience and knowledge of the patient, to determine dosages and the best treatment for each individual patient. Neither the Publisher nor the authors assumes any liability for any injury and/or damage to persons or property arising from this publication.

The Publisher

ELSEVIER your source for books,
journals and multimedia
in the health sciences
www.elsevierhealth.com

The
Publisher's
policy is to use
**paper manufactured
from sustainable forests**

Printed in China

Contents

Acknowledgements

We would like to thank the following people for their contribution to the book:

Jason Smith, Sue Masel, Matt Masel and **Lawrie Hirst** for their careful proof reading and excellent suggestions; at Elsevier, **Michael Parkinson** for picking up the book and **Hannah Kenner** for her energy and professionalism in its production; and my wife **Kath** for her endless patience, support and encouragement.

Anthony Pane

Mae and **Reg** for their continuous support and **Astrid** for her patience; **Ray MacLeod**, Medical Photographer, West of England Eye Unit, for his hard work in helping with the photographs.

Peter Simcock

Introduction

As a medical student, hospital doctor or general practitioner you can't be expected to know everything. Ophthalmology is only one of many specialties, each with its own list of rare and unpleasant diseases you are sternly told you 'can't afford to miss!' You usually have minimal examination time and little or no equipment. Despite this, many of your patients have eye complaints and rely on you for appropriate management. What do you do?

As an optometry student or optometrist you spend your life examining eyes, most of which are normal apart from refractive error. However, a few of your patients will present to you with potentially blinding or even life-threatening disease, which will have serious consequences if missed. How do you identify these patients and what do you do then?

This book is a symptom-based guide to ophthalmology for the non-ophthalmologist. Many eye books list disease by anatomical site, but patients don't present saying 'I have a disease of my optic nerve'. Instead, they walk into your office and complain of blurred vision. Each of the main chapters in this book concentrates on a different presenting symptom, and contains:

- An *overview* of the problem.
- *Critical points* highlighting important management issues.
- *Diagnostic flowcharts.*
- An *approach* to use for the patient sitting before you, including questions to ask and signs to look for.
- A brief discussion of the symptoms, signs and management of the relevant common eye *diseases*.

Some chapters include special features:

- *Chapter 1* Staying out of trouble with eyes – contains practical guidelines to help you avoid serious mistakes in your everyday practice.

- *Chapter 2* How to examine an eye patient – outlines a time-efficient way to assess eye patients.
- *Chapter 10* Who needs screening for eye disease? – a guide to which of your patients require regular eye screening.
- *Chapter 11* Basic eye procedures – details common practical eye procedures.

Ophthalmic diagnosis is often difficult, even with the luxury of time and the appropriate technology. However, even a brief history and examination with basic equipment can be enough to identify the general nature of most eye diseases. We hope this book helps.

How to use this book

Medical students: read the chapters in order.

General practitioners:
● If you're already good at eye examination: skip Chapter 2.
● Short of time? Read Chapters 1 and 10 then have a look at the overview, flowcharts and photographs in the other chapters.
● Keep the book handy for quick reference in the clinic.

Emergency department doctors:
● If you're already good at eye examination: skip Chapter 2.
● Short of time? Chapters 1, 3, 4, 5 and 11 are particularly important for you.

Optometry students – first year: read the chapters in order.

Optometrists and senior optometry students:
● Skip Chapters 2 and 11.
● Short of time? Read Chapters 1 and 10 then have a look at the overview, flowcharts and photographs in the other chapters.
● Keep the book handy for quick reference in the clinic.

Please note:
● There are thousands of eye diseases, about which millions of pages have been written. A brief book such as this relies on massive over-simplification and there are many rare eye diseases not discussed here at all.
● Writing for such a wide audience means starting 'from the basics'; we acknowledge that many readers will already be highly knowledgeable about some of the areas covered (more advanced texts are suggested in the Further Reading).
● This book is not intended to be a substitute for thorough clinical training. The best way to learn ophthalmic diagnosis and

management is by sitting in clinic with an experienced ophthalmologist.

● In this book, 'ophthalmic referral' or 'ophthalmic assessment' means referral to an ophthalmologist (eye surgeon) or ophthalmic emergency department.

● Often, 'real life' cases aren't as clear-cut as on the printed page; **if in doubt, refer**.

STAYING OUT OF TROUBLE WITH EYES

CHAPTER CONTENTS

OVERVIEW

No-one will care much if you 'miss' chronic allergic conjunctivitis or cataracts – the patient will eventually be diagnosed by someone else, and no harm done. However, if you misdiagnose iritis as conjunctivitis, and give antibiotic drops for a month when the patient should have been urgently referred, the chance to save vision might be lost. Likewise, if you post a written referral for a patient who has presented to you with sudden-onset double vision, they have a small chance of dying from rupture of an undiagnosed cerebral aneurysm while waiting for their ophthalmology appointment. How can these tragic errors, which can be made by very diligent doctors and optometrists, be avoided?

Fortunately, observing a few simple guidelines increases the chance of your eye patients (and you) avoiding trouble. These 'critical points' are based on the common mistakes made by practitioners referring to eye emergency departments and outpatients. These points also appear at the start of the relevant chapters.

AVOIDING THE MOST COMMON MISTAKES OF ALL DOCTORS

- Please *do not*, as a reflex, prescribe antibiotic drops for all patients with a red eye and tell them to come back in a week or to go to the hospital if they get worse. Although this will satisfy the patient's initial demand for 'treatment', the drops are no good for a serious eye condition: they can interfere with microbiological investigations (if the patient really does have an eye infection) and, more importantly, they can seriously delay referral, which might cost a patient his or her sight.
- The only time you should prescribe antibiotic drops or ointment is for bacterial conjunctivitis: *two* red eyes, *pus-like* discharge, *normal* vision, *no* pain or photophobia. Red eye(s) from some other cause will either resolve with no treatment (e.g. viral conjunctivitis), require a different treatment (e.g. allergic conjunctivitis) or require urgent referral (e.g. iritis or infectious corneal ulcer).

OPTOMETRISTS

- If a patient's vision is worse than that expected from an examination of the eye, suspect that there is something *behind* the eye (sometimes a tumour compressing the optic nerve or chiasm). Patients with pituitary tumours compressing the anterior visual pathway most commonly present first to optometrists, complaining of blurred vision or field loss.

- **Checking visual fields to confrontation and performing the 'swinging torch' test for relative afferent pupillary defect (RAPD) should be part of the routine examination of every new patient complaining of blurred vision.** These tests only take 30 seconds but are often the only way to clinically detect serious visual pathway pathology.

How to examine an eye patient **Critical points**

- **Most eye diseases cannot be definitively diagnosed without a slit lamp microscope examination.**

- **The basic examination of every eye patient should include:**
  - visual acuity testing
  - confrontation visual field testing
  - the 'swinging torch' test for relative afferent pupillary defect
  - examination of the front of the eye (ideally with a slit lamp microscope)
  - examination of the optic discs and retina (with the ophthalmoscope or, ideally, with a slit lamp retinal lens)
  - measurement of intraocular pressure (if available).

- **Every general practice should have:**
  - a distance visual acuity chart
  - a bright torch with a detachable blue filter
  - some type of magnifier for anterior segment examination
  - a working direct ophthalmoscope
  - fluorescein eye drops to detect corneal ulcers
  - tropicamide dilating drops to use before ophthalmoscopy.

Visual loss *Critical points*

- **Any patient with unexplained visual loss requires ophthalmic referral.**

- **If visual loss is sudden or rapidly progressive, referral must be *urgent* (ideally, the patient should be seen the same day).**

- **Beware of 'worse than expected' vision:** a level of vision that is worse than would be expected from visible intraocular disease can indicate the presence of optic nerve or brain visual pathway disease.

- **Not all visual loss is caused by eye disease:** the first symptom of orbit or brain tumours and strokes can be blurred vision.

- **Serious eye or brain disease is likely if a patient with blurred vision also has one or more of the following *symptoms*:**
  - unexplained eye pain
  - sensitivity to light (photophobia)
  - distortion of vision (metamorphopsia)
  - flashes of light
  - new-onset floating spots
  - loss of part of the visual field
  - symptoms of temporal arteritis (in patients over 50; see p. 216).

- **Serious eye or brain disease is likely if a patient with blurred vision also has one or more of these *signs*:**
  - red eye
  - visual field defect
  - relative afferent pupil defect (see p. 25)
  - abnormality of the cornea, iris or pupil
  - loss of the red reflex
  - optic disc swelling or pallor.

The red eye *Critical points*

- **All cases of red eye of unknown cause with decreased vision, pain or photophobia require urgent (same-day) referral to an ophthalmologist or ophthalmic emergency department.** Do not prescribe any treatment for these patients before referral – this wastes time and can interfere with investigations.

- **Do not call every red eye 'conjunctivitis'!** There are many other causes of red eye, many of them serious and requiring urgent treatment by an ophthalmologist.

- **The only time you should prescribe antibiotic drops or ointment is for bacterial conjunctivitis:** *two* red eyes, *pus-like* discharge, *normal* vision, *no* pain or photophobia. Red eye(s) of other causes will either resolve with no treatment (e.g. viral conjunctivitis), require a different treatment (e.g. allergic conjunctivitis), or require urgent referral (e.g. iritis or infectious corneal ulcer).

- **Never prescribe steroid or antibiotic–steroid eye drops** unless asked to by an ophthalmologist – serious damage to the eye can occur.

- **A newborn baby with red eyes and eye discharge** has sight- and life-threatening infection (ophthalmia neonatorum; see p. 105) until proven otherwise, and requires urgent ophthalmic review.

Eye trauma *Critical points*

- **If a high-velocity foreign body has hit the eye, consider that it is *in* the eye until proven otherwise** (by X-ray or CT scan, and careful ophthalmic examination).

- **If you suspect your patient has a possible penetrating eye injury, an urgent telephone consultation with an ophthalmologist is required to plan emergency transfer and surgery.** Keep the patient nil by mouth, place a hard shield (not a soft patch) over the eye, and give antiemetics and analgesia as required. *Continues*

Eye trauma *Critical points—cont'd*

- **Any patient with head or facial trauma (including a 'black eye') should have a basic eye examination** to exclude serious eye injuries. Every patient with a 'black eye' has serious underlying eye trauma until proven otherwise.

- **Alkali and acid burns** to the eyes are potentially sight-threatening and require urgent thorough eye irrigation (water or saline) for 30 minutes, followed by urgent ophthalmic opinion.

'Turned eye' in children **Critical points**

- **A child of any age with strabismus ('turned eye') has a sight- or life-threatening condition until proven otherwise and needs prompt referral.** Childhood tumours of the brain and eye often present with a turned eye.

- **Never 'observe' a child with strabismus** – it is very rare for a child to 'grow out of it'. Delay in ophthalmic referral can result in permanent visual loss from amblyopia ('lazy eye').

Double vision in adults **Critical points**

- **New-onset double vision** in a patient of any age is a life-threatening cerebral aneurysm until proven otherwise – **all require urgent (same-day) ophthalmic referral.**

- **Never prescribe spectacle prism** for double vision of unknown cause unless the patient has been assessed by an ophthalmologist. Brain tumours are a common cause of gradual-onset diplopia.

- **If a patient over 50 has transient or persisting double vision, ask about symptoms of temporal arteritis (see p. 216).**

Abnormal eye or eyelid appearance **Critical points**

- **Every neonate should have their red reflexes checked** with a direct ophthalmoscope in a dark room, as part of their routine first physical examination.

- **A child with an absent red reflex or white pupil** has a retinoblastoma or cataract until proven otherwise – refer urgently.

- **A child or adult with severely swollen red eyelids on one side** has orbital cellulitis until proven otherwise – this is a sight- and life-threatening medical emergency.

- **If the patient can't blink, the cornea is in danger** – patients with facial nerve palsies or major facial burns need intensive lubricant eye ointment treatment, plus urgent ophthalmic consultation to prevent corneal ulceration.

- **Swollen optic discs can be the only sign of a brain tumour** – for this reason, every patient with headaches requires ophthalmoscopy as part of the routine examination, and urgent referral if disc swelling is found.

Watery, itchy or gritty eyes **Critical points**

- **Any patient with unexplained foreign body sensation requires ophthalmic referral** (urgently if there is also blurred vision, pain or photophobia).

- **A baby with watery eye(s)** probably has harmless nasolacrimal duct obstruction. However, if **photophobia, corneal clouding or corneal enlargement** are present the child should be suspected of having **congenital glaucoma** and be referred urgently.

Other eye symptoms **Critical points**

- **New-onset 'flashes' and/or 'floaters' in one eye are a retinal detachment until proven otherwise – refer urgently.**

- **Not all flashing lights and headache is migraine –** occasionally, occipital tumours and vertebrobasilar transient ischaemic attacks can also cause flashes.

- **Every patient with blurred vision or headaches requires confrontation visual field testing.** This might be the only way to detect a brain tumour (e.g. pituitary tumour causing bitemporal hemianopia).

- **Visual field loss always requires ophthalmic assessment** (urgently if of sudden onset or if visual pathway disease is suspected) – it could be due to disease in the retina, optic nerve(s), or brain.

- **Sudden-onset visual distortion (metamorphopsia)** is likely to be due to acute macular disease – refer urgently.

- **Temporal arteritis should be considered in every patient aged over 50 with one or more of:**
  - transient or persisting vision loss or double vision
  - new headaches, scalp tenderness on hair brushing, jaw muscle ache on chewing food, ear or neck pain, weight loss, fatigue, muscle aches
  - temporal arteries that are tender to palpation and/or not pulsatile
  - if suspicious: urgent referral.

Who needs screening for eye disease? **Critical points**

- **All patients with diabetes require a careful retinal examination at diagnosis, and then yearly for the rest of their lives.** A direct ophthalmoscope examination is not adequate for screening as it can miss early or moderate diabetic maculopathy.

- **All adults over age 40 should have a glaucoma screening test (intraocular pressure and optic disc examination) by their optometrist every 2 years for the rest of their lives.** Patients who have close relatives with glaucoma should obtain ophthalmic advice regarding the age at which screening should begin.

- Certain other patients benefit from routine eye screening – see Chapter 10.

HOW TO EXAMINE
AN EYE PATIENT

CHAPTER CONTENTS

OVERVIEW

This chapter outlines a method of history taking and examination that will identify the general nature of most eye diseases. Crucial points in the history and examination for each major eye symptom are also emphasised in the 'Approach' section in the individual chapters of this book. *Please skip this chapter if you're already good at eye examination.*

How to examine an eye patient *Critical points*

- **Most eye diseases cannot be diagnosed definitively without a slit lamp microscope examination.**

- **The basic examination of every eye patient should include:**
  - visual acuity testing
  - confrontation visual field testing
  - the 'swinging torch test' for relative afferent pupillary defect (RAPD)
  - examination of the front of the eye (ideally with a slit lamp microscope)
  - examination of the optic discs and retina (with the ophthalmoscope or, ideally, with a slit lamp retinal lens)
  - measurement of intraocular pressure (if available).

- **Every general practice should have:**
  - a distance visual acuity (VA) chart
  - a bright torch with a detachable blue filter
  - some type of magnifier for anterior segment examination
  - a working direct ophthalmoscope
  - fluorescein eyedrops to detect corneal ulcers
  - tropicamide dilating drops to use before ophthalmoscopy.

THE VISUAL SYSTEM (Fig. 2.1)

A good (but not strictly optically correct) analogy is that **the eye is like a camera** (Fig. 2.2):

- There is a clear sheet of glass at the front (the **cornea**). The curved cornea contributes most of the eye's 'fixed' focusing power.

- The camera can take sharp pictures of both near and distant objects by changing the focus of the lens. The eye's **lens** lies behind the iris; the shape of the lens is altered when the ciliary muscle in the ciliary body contracts to allow the focus to be changed.

- The focused light forms an inverted picture on the light-sensitive film, the **retina**. The retina is a thin sheet lining the inside of the back of the eyeball. It contains millions of light-sensitive cells (rods and cones) plus a complex circuitry of other nerve cells. The most sensitive central area of the retina (the part we use for reading and colour vision) is called the **macula**.

- An adjustable aperture controls the amount of light entering the camera. The eye's aperture is the black hole (**pupil**) in the adjustable diaphragm (the coloured **iris**).

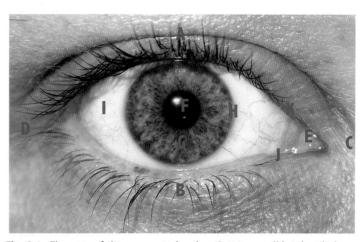

Fig. 2.1 The parts of the eye – anterior view. **A**, upper eyelid and eyelashes; **B**, lower eyelid and eyelashes; **C**, medial canthus; **D**, lateral canthus; **E**, caruncle; **F**, pupil (behind the clear cornea); **G**, iris (behind the clear cornea); **H**, limbus; **I**, white sclera, covered by clear conjunctiva; **J**, position of inferior lacrimal punctum; **K**, position of superior lacrimal punctum.

- These fragile 'working parts' are surrounded by a tough camera case (the white **sclera**). This completely surrounds the eyeball, except where the optic nerve comes out at the back and where the clear cornea sits at the front.
- The retina (the eye's 'film') rests on a black, light-absorbent platform: between the light-sensitive retina and the outer sclera is a layer of blood vessels and pigment called the **choroid**. The choroid's function is to keep the very fragile retina supplied with nutrients, and to catch stray light within the eye with its dark pigment.

Unlike a camera, however, the eye is filled with **fluid**. There are two fluid spaces in the eye:

1. The **anterior chamber** – between the coloured iris and the clear cornea: this is filled with a clear, watery fluid called **aqueous**. Aqueous is produced continuously by the ciliary body, and is continuously drained out of the eye by structures in the 'angle', where the clear cornea, coloured iris and white sclera meet. A block in this fluid drainage process causes high pressure in the eye (glaucoma).
2. The **vitreous cavity** – between the lens (which is just behind the iris) and the retina: this contains a clear jelly called **vitreous**. Vitreous is a firm jelly early in life but breaks down later in life into solid and liquid parts (patients often see the solid parts as 'floaters').

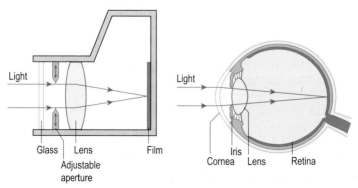

Fig. 2.2 The eye as a camera.

Visual information from the retina needs to be interpreted in the brain. The optic nerve is a single 'cable' of more than one million nerve fibres. It carries information about the 'picture' taken by the retina to the brain. The exit point of the optic nerve from the back of the eye can be seen with an ophthalmoscope as the circular optic disc (or optic nerve head) (Fig. 2.3). Nerve impulses are relayed through the visual pathways of the brain.

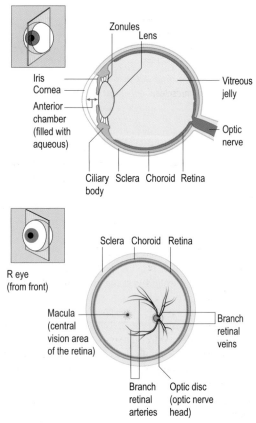

Fig. 2.3 The eye in cross-section.

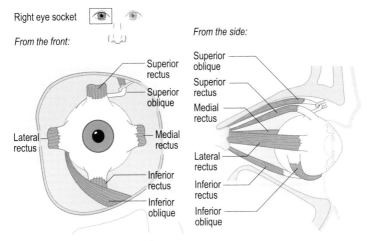

Fig. 2.4 The extraocular muscles.

The eyes need to be able to move in the head:

● Six **extraocular muscles** (Fig. 2.4) attached to each eyeball move the eyes (usually together) to look at objects of interest – these muscles are:

   ▶ four 'rectus' muscles: superior, inferior, lateral and medial (attached to the sclera of the eyeball in the positions suggested by their names)

   ▶ two 'oblique' muscles: superior and inferior.

● The main actions of these muscles (Fig. 2.5) are:

   ▶ medial rectus – rotates the eyeball towards the nose (adduction)

   ▶ lateral rectus – rotates the eyeball towards the ear (abduction)

   ▶ superior rectus – rotates the eyeball up (elevation)

   ▶ inferior rectus – rotates the eyeball down (depression)

   ▶ superior oblique – rolls the eyeball inwards (intorsion)

   ▶ inferior oblique – rolls the eyeball outwards (extorsion).

● All the muscles are supplied by the third cranial nerve (oculomotor nerve) except for:

   ▶ the superior oblique, which is supplied by the fourth (trochlear) nerve

   ▶ the lateral rectus, which is supplied by the sixth (abducens) nerve.

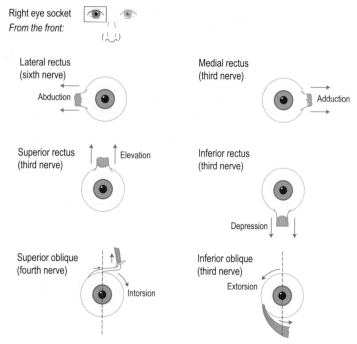

Fig. 2.5 Actions of the extraocular muscles.

The eyes need to be protected and lubricated:

- Each eyeball sits in a protective bony 'eye socket' in the face, the **orbit**. This contains the eyeball, optic nerve, extraocular muscles, nerves and blood vessels, and cushioning fat.

- The surface of the eyes are continually lubricated by the blinking of the **eyelids**, which keep the sensitive corneal surface wet with tears.

- The eyelids contain a backbone of white connective tissue, the **tarsal plate**, which accounts for the ability to evert ('flip') the top eyelids over.

- Blinking and eyelid closure is performed by the **orbicularis muscle**, which is supplied by the seventh (facial) nerve.

- Eyelid opening (raising the upper eyelid) is performed by the **levator muscle** ('levator palpebrae superioris'), which is supplied by the third (oculomotor) nerve.

- Where the upper and lower eyelids meet is called the **canthus**:
  - the meeting point towards the nose is the medial (or inner) canthus
  - the meeting point towards the ear is the lateral (or outer) canthus
  - the fleshy pink triangle of tissue between the lids at the medial canthus is the **caruncle**.
- The outer surface of the white sclera and the inner surface of the eyelids is lined by a thin, transparent, protective skin called the **conjunctiva**.
- Tears are produced by the **lacrimal gland** (in the orbit just above the eye) (Fig. 2.6) and are drained by the **lacrimal drainage system**, a system of tubes consisting of:
  - the lacrimal punctae (two small holes, one in each of the upper and lower eyelids near the nose, where tears enter the drainage system)
  - the lacrimal canaliculae (tubes running from the punctae through the eyelids towards the nose)
  - the lacrimal sac (in the bony wall of the nose)
  - the nasolacrimal duct (a tube from the sac through the bone of the nose wall that opens into the nose, which is why crying causes the nose to run).

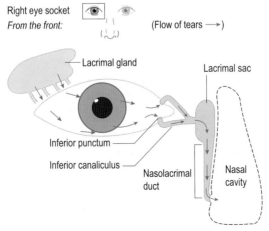

Right eye socket
From the front:

(Flow of tears ⟶)

Lacrimal gland

Lacrimal sac

Inferior punctum

Inferior canaliculus

Nasolacrimal duct

Nasal cavity

Fig. 2.6 The lacrimal gland and lacrimal drainage system.

THE VISUAL PATHWAY OF THE BRAIN

Visual information from the two eyes passes from the optic nerves at the front of the brain to the visual cortex at the back of the brain (Fig. 2.7), via the:

- optic nerve
- optic chiasm
- optic tract
- lateral geniculate nucleus (LGN)
- optic radiation.

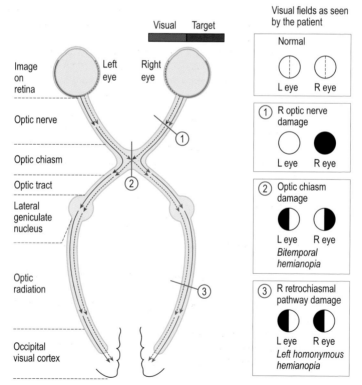

Fig. 2.7 View of eyes and brain from above: the visual pathways.

- primary visual cortex in the occipital lobe
- higher visual cortical areas.

The optic chiasm is the X-shaped structure at the base of the brain formed by the meeting of the two optic nerves. An important rearrangement of the optic nerve fibres occurs in the chiasm.

Anterior to (in front of) the chiasm

Each optic nerve carries information about the whole visual field of the eye to which it is attached. Damage to one optic nerve thus causes visual field loss limited to the eye on the same side.

In the chiasm

Half of the fibres from each optic nerve cross to the other side of the brain, as shown in Fig. 2.7:

- fibres arising from the nasal (inner) half of the retina of each eye **cross** to the other side, carrying visual information from the **temporal (outer) half of the visual field of each eye**.
- the other retinal fibres pass through uncrossed.

Because of this arrangement, an injury to the centre of the chiasm (e.g. compression from a pituitary tumour) will damage the crossing fibres first and cause loss of part or all of the temporal (outer) half of the visual field of each eye. This is called a **bitemporal hemianopia**.

Posterior to (behind) the chiasm

The 'retrochiasmal' visual pathway on each side carries information about the **opposite** half of the visual field of **both** eyes back to the visual cortex, e.g. the left-sided retrochiasmal pathway carries information about the right half of the left eye's visual field and the right half of the right eye's visual field.

Injury to the visual pathway behind the chiasm on one side will therefore cause loss of some or all of the opposite visual hemifields of both eyes. This is called a **homonymous hemianopia**.

All this is important because *the pattern of visual field loss can help you localise where disease is in the brain.*

HISTORY

Asking patients in detail about their eye complaints will often be very helpful in diagnosing the problem.

PRESENTING COMPLAINT

- What is the main problem, e.g. blurred vision, pain, redness, irritation?
- Is it in one or both eyes?
  - *Caution*: patients with bilateral visual field loss (e.g. from a stroke or brain tumour) might misinterpret the vision problem as being present only in the eye with the more prominent field loss.
- Rapidity of onset: was onset sudden or gradual?
- Pain: is there a scratchy sensation at the front of the eye, or deep aching pain inside the eye?
- If the problem resulted from an injury, what was the mechanism of injury?

SPECIFIC QUESTIONS

See the relevant chapters for more details:
- Specific questions for painless visual loss without history of trauma:
  - new onset flashes and/or floaters? (possible retinal detachment)
  - loss of part of the visual field? (retinal detachment, other retinal disease, optic nerve or brain disease)
  - distortion of straight lines? (metamorphopsia – macular disease).
- If the patient is over age 50, are there any headaches/scalp tenderness/jaw muscle ache on chewing? (these are the symptoms of temporal arteritis; see p. 216 for other symptoms)
- Specific questions for red eye:
  - was there an injury?
  - is it painful?
  - blurred vision?
  - photophobia? (i.e. sensitive to light?)

PREVIOUS OPHTHALMIC HISTORY

- Contact lens wear? (increased risk of corneal infections).
- Previous intraocular operations? (increased risk of retinal detachment).

PREVIOUS MEDICAL AND SURGICAL HISTORY

In particular, find out about:

- Diabetes (diabetic retinopathy – make sure regular ophthalmic screening has been arranged).
- Hypertension (increased risk of retinal vascular occlusions).
- Grave's disease (hyperthyroidism – can cause thyroid eye disease).
- Carotid stenosis, atrial fibrillation, heart murmurs, artificial heart valves (emboli to retina causing branch retinal artery occlusion).

MEDICATIONS

- Is the patient taking any eye medications?
- Is the patient taking any medications that can cause eye problems? (see Chapter 10 for medications that require regular eye screening).

FAMILY HISTORY

- Patients with a first-degree relative with glaucoma or retinal detachment are at increased risk of developing the condition themselves.

EXAMINATION

Step-wise in the following order:
1. visual acuity
2. visual fields to confrontation
3. eye movements (if the patient is a child with 'turned eye' or an adult with double vision)
4. pupils and 'swinging torch test'
5. torch examination of the lids and eyes
6. slit lamp examination (if available)
7. intraocular pressure testing (if available)
8. ophthalmoscopy
9. other tests if necessary.

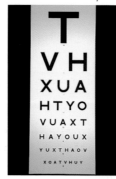
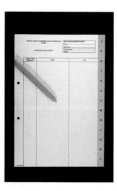

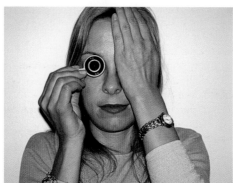

Fig. 2.8 Testing visual acuity. Top left, visual acuity chart; top right, a home-made pinhole; bottom, using a commercial pinhole.

VISUAL ACUITY (VA) (Fig. 2.8)

- Position the patient 6 metres (20 feet) from a Snellen (or equivalent) visual acuity eye chart (Fig. 2.8 top left).
- Examine one eye at a time.
- If the patient needs glasses or contact lenses for clear distance vision (e.g. watching television, driving), use these.
- If vision is poor, see if it improves with the glasses off and the patient looking through a 'pinhole' with each eye in turn (Fig. 2.8 bottom). Use a commercial pinhole or make your own by pushing a hole in a sheet of paper with a pen (Fig. 2.8 top right). This roughly corrects any refractive error present (it might also improve vision in some cases of cataract or corneal scar).
- Note the visual acuity, e.g. if the patient can read the '12' line with the right eye, write 'right 6/12' (said 'six twelve').
- If the patient can't read any letters at all, can he or she:
  - count fingers ('CF')
  - see hand movements ('HM')
  - perceive light ('PL'); or does the patient have no perception of light ('NPL')?

VISUAL FIELDS

Testing the patient's left visual field to confrontation (Fig. 2.9):
- Sit directly in front of the patient with your eyes at the same level as theirs, about an arm's length away.
- Close your left eye.
- Ask the patient to cover their right eye with their right hand and to stare into your right eye.
- Compare the patient's peripheral visual field to your own: hold up one, two or five fingers midway between yourself and the patient in the mid-peripheral visual field (so you can see them yourself). Ask the patient how many fingers you are holding up.
- Repeat for all four quadrants of the visual field (upper right, upper left, lower right, lower left).
- Repeat for the right eye.

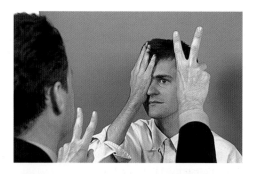

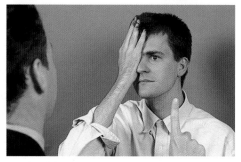

Fig. 2.9 Testing visual fields to confrontation.

EYE MOVEMENTS

These only need to be tested if the patient is complaining of double vision, or if one eye is 'turned' (see p. 133 for how to test).

PUPILS AND THE 'SWINGING TORCH' TEST

Answer three separate questions:
1. Are both pupils the same size?
2. Do they both react briskly to light?
3. Is there a relative afferent pupillary defect (RAPD)?

The 'swinging torch' test for a relative afferent pupillary defect (*RAPD*) (Fig. 2.10)

This is a very important test and should be performed on every patient complaining of blurred vision, field loss, flashes or floaters:

- Dim or turn off the room lights.
- Use the brightest torch or ophthalmoscope light you have.
- Ask the patient to stare at a target in the distance (e.g. on the opposite wall).
- Swing the torch repeatedly back and forth between the two eyes (2 seconds on each eye) – hold the torch slightly below the eyes, so as not to interrupt the line of sight.
- A normal response is for each pupil to **constrict** (become slightly smaller) when the torch is shone on it.
- A relative afferent pupil defect (abnormal response) is present when the torch is swung from one eye to the other and the pupil of the illuminated eye dilates (becomes larger) instead of constricting as is normal.
- You are looking at the **dynamic movement** of the pupil (whether it constricts or dilates) in this test, and not at the final pupil size.
- **The presence of a relative afferent pupil defect alerts you that your patient has serious *widespread retinal disease* (e.g. retinal detachment) or *optic nerve disease* in the eye with the relative afferent pupil defect.**
- Bilateral but asymmetric retinal or optic nerve disease will cause a RAPD in the 'worse' eye.
- Bilateral retinal or optic nerve disease that is equally bad in both eyes will *not* cause a RAPD.
- As a general rule, a relative afferent pupil defect is *never* caused by:
  - corneal disease
  - cataract (even if advanced and unilateral)
  - vitreous haemorrhage (without retinal detachment)
  - macular disease.

TORCH EXAMINATION OF THE EYELIDS AND EYES

This is useful to do even if you have a slit lamp. With the room lights on, have a careful look at the eye and eyelids with your torch (or with a hand-held magnifying lens if you have one).

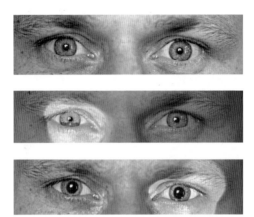

Fig. 2.10 A left relative afferent pupil defect (RAPD) demonstrated on the 'swinging torch' test. Top, both pupils are equal size in normal room lighting; middle, room lights are dimmed and patient asked to look into distance, the right pupil constricts when the torch is shone on it; bottom, the left pupil dilates when the torch is swung from the right eye to the left. The torch is then swung back to the right pupil, which constricts again; then back to the left, which dilates again; this can be repeated as often as you wish.

With white torch light

- Is the eye red?
- Does it look like the other eye?
- Is the cornea clear (as is normal), cloudy or is there an ulcer?
- Is there visible blood (hyphaema) or pus (hypopyon) in the anterior chamber?
- Are the eyelids normal?

With blue torch light plus fluorescein drops (Fig. 2.11)

- Fluorescein is a yellow or orange eyedrop that fluoresces when a blue light is shone on it.
- This fluorescence shows up scratches, abrasions or ulcers on the surface of the cornea and conjunctiva that might not be easily visible with white light alone.
- There is no need for a commercial blue filter – a piece of blue cellophane held over the end of your torch with an elastic band will work just as well.

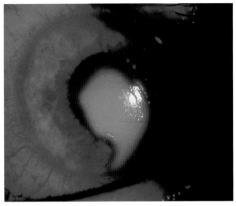

Fig. 2.11 Corneal abrasion viewed with blue light, after a drop of fluorescein was put in the eye.

- Don't use fluorescein (or any eyedrops) if you suspect a penetrating eye injury.

Eyelid eversion

Eyelid eversion is necessary if:
- The patient complains of foreign body sensation and you can't see any abnormality with the torch and/or slit lamp.
- The patient has lost a contact lens (it could be under the top lid).
- You are irrigating the eye after a chemical burn.
  Eyelid eversion should *not* be done if a penetrating eye injury is suspected.

LOWER LID

Simply pull the lower lid down as much as possible, looking in the inferior conjunctival fornix (recess) for a foreign body.

UPPER LID (Fig. 2.12)

This needs practice:
- Ask the patient to keep both eyes open and to look down.
- Grasp the upper lid lashes firmly between your left thumb and forefinger and pull the lid away from the eye.

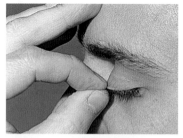
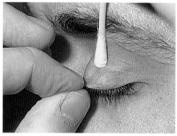

Fig. 2.12 Upper eyelid eversion.

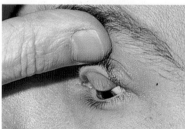

- Holding a cotton bud vertically between your right thumb and index finger, press down vertically into the eyelid about 1 cm superior to the lid margin.
- Flip the lid over by continuing to push down with the cotton bud while pulling the lashes upwards with your left hand.
- Once the lid is flipped over, keep holding the lid margin with your left hand and withdraw the cotton bud.
- Now inspect the inner surface of the lid.

SLIT LAMP EXAMINATION

The slit lamp is a binocular microscope for looking at the eye (Fig. 2.13). It allows high-magnification viewing of the cornea, conjunctiva, sclera, anterior chamber, iris, lens and anterior vitreous. With the use of hand-held retinal lenses (Fig. 2.13 right), it also allows magnified stereoscopic views of the posterior vitreous, optic disc and retina.

- ***It is impossible to definitively diagnose most eye diseases without a slit lamp examination***

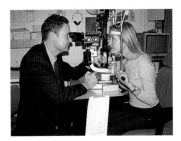 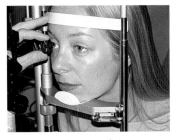

Fig. 2.13 Using the slit lamp. Left: viewing the anterior part of the eye; right: viewing the optic disc and retina with a retinal lens.

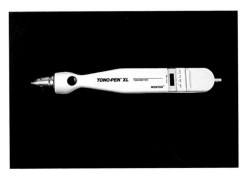

Fig. 2.14 The Tonopen.

⬤ If you are a doctor in an emergency department with a slit lamp, make sure someone shows you how to use it.

INTRAOCULAR PRESSURE TESTING

If the intraocular pressure (IOP) is too high (as in glaucoma), the eye can be damaged. Three major types of instruments (tonometers) are currently used to measure intraocular pressure:

⬤ Tonopen (Fig. 2.14): this is the ideal tonometer for hospital emergency departments and rural general practitioners. It is easy to use, portable and quite accurate.

⬤ Air-puff tonometer: many optometrists use this tonometer.

⬤ Goldmann tonometer: this is the most difficult tonometer to use, but the most accurate. It is a small prism device fitted on the slit lamp and requires the use of blue light and fluorescein drops.

OPHTHALMOSCOPY WITH THE DIRECT OPHTHALMOSCOPE

The direct ophthalmoscope has a very small field of view (it allows a view of only a tiny part of the back of the eye at any one time). For this reason it is good for looking at the optic disc (if dilating drops have been used) but does *not* allow accurate diagnosis of retinal disease.

A slit lamp with a hand-held retinal lens or an indirect ophthalmoscope is required to diagnose most retinal diseases.

Dilating drops

Ophthalmoscopy is much easier and more accurate if the patient's pupils are first dilated. The most common dilating drop is tropicamide 1%:

- Use one drop in each eye.
- Wait 15 minutes and repeat if dilation is not adequate.
- Warn the patient:
  - the effects will take 8 hours to wear off; in that time vision will be 'bright' and blurry; the patient should not drive
  - to return immediately if severe eye pain or a red eye develops: dilating drops can (*very rarely*) precipitate acute glaucoma.
- Tropicamide is not suitable for children; in general don't dilate children at all (leave this to the examining ophthalmologist).

Using the direct ophthalmoscope

- If the patient has glasses, remove them. If you have glasses, leave them on.
- Darken the room.
- First check the red reflex:
  - place the lens wheel of the ophthalmoscope on '0' (no corrective lens)
  - turn the ophthalmoscope light on to moderate intensity
  - sit or stand an arm's length away from the patient
  - look through the ophthalmoscope at the patient
  - ask the patient to look at the light
  - a normal red reflex response is seen as a diffuse red or orange glow in the pupil.
- Then examine the optic disc and retina (preferably after dilating drops):

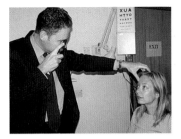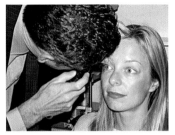

Fig. 2.15 Using the direct ophthalmoscope. Left, checking the red reflex; right, viewing the optic disc and retina.

- ask the patient (who is seated) to stare straight ahead at a target on the wall, and to keep staring there even if your head gets in the way
- to examine the patient's right eye, close your left eye and hold the ophthalmoscope up to your right eye with your right hand
- to orient yourself, rest your left hand at arm's length on the right side of the patient's forehead (Fig. 2.15 left)
- stand directly in front of the patient, then take a step to your left
- looking through the ophthalmoscope the whole time, with the light shining on the patient's right eye, slowly approach the patient's right eye until your heads are very close (Fig. 2.15 right)
- view the optic disc (it is not in the centre of the retina but slightly towards the nasal side)
- turn the focus wheel with your right index finger until the image is sharply in focus
- assess the disc carefully
- follow the major retinal vessels in turn away from the disc
- to assess the peripheral retina as much as possible (only a very limited retinal examination is possible with this instrument due to its very small field of view), ask the patient to look up, down, left and right while viewing.
- Finally, to view the macula (central area of the retina), ask the patient to stare directly into your light.

Normal optic disc appearance

The optic disc is visible as a flat circular area situated slightly to the nasal side of the centre of the back of the eye. The main retinal vessels emerge from the disc.

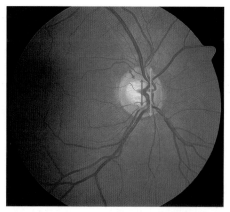

Fig. 2.16 Normal optic disc. Green arrow, total disc height; red arrow, central 'cup'; blue arrow, 'rim'. The cup–disc ratio = the height of the green arrow divided by the height of the red arrow = approximately 0.5 in this case.

- To find the disc with the direct ophthalmoscope, find a retinal vessel and trace it back to the disc.
- The parts of the disc are:
  - a flat outer pink 'rim'
  - a central excavated paler 'cup'.
- The 'cup-disc ratio' (Fig. 2.16):
  - this is the ratio of the vertical height of the central cup to the total vertical height of the disc, expressed as a decimal fraction, e.g. if the cup is half as high as the total disc height, the cup–disc ratio is 0.5
  - discs that are abnormally 'cupped' (as in glaucoma) have an enlarged and deepened central cup and a cup–disc ratio that is usually greater than 0.5.

Normal retinal appearance

- The normal retina has an orange or pink colour in Caucasians and a darker colour in dark-skinned patients.
- The centre of the retina is the macula. This is visible as a darker area (Fig. 2.17) that is brought into view if the patient looks directly at your ophthalmoscope light.

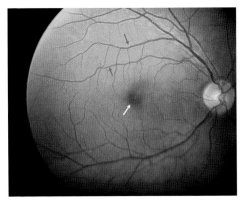

Fig. 2.17 Normal appearance of the retina (this is a much wider field of view than that obtainable with the direct ophthalmoscope). Yellow arrow, macula; red arrow, superotemporal branch retinal artery; blue arrow, superotemporal branch retinal vein.

- The normal macula is featureless apart from a central spot-like or ring-like reflection of your light.
- Four main retinal vascular 'arcades' radiate out from the optic disc, each consisting of a branch retinal vein and a branch retinal artery:
  - superotemporal and inferotemporal (which curve above and below the macula)
  - superonasal and inferonasal (on the other side of the disc from the macula).

OTHER TESTS

Other tests are not performed routinely but might be needed for particular problems.

Amsler grid

This is a small sheet of paper with a grid of black lines on it (Fig. 2.18). It is used for testing the central visual field, most commonly when macular disease (e.g. age-related macular degeneration) is suspected. To use the grid, ask the patient to:

- Put on their reading glasses, cover one eye, and hold the grid about 30 cm away.

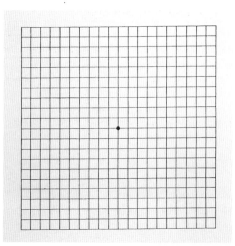

Fig. 2.18 The Amsler grid.

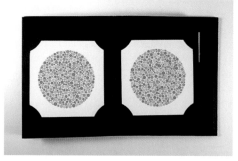

Fig. 2.19 Ishihara plate book.

- Look at the central dot of the grid.
- Now ask: 'do all the lines look straight and clear, or are some of the lines curved or missing?'
- Significant macular disease is likely if the patient reports that lines are wavy or there are blank spots on the grid.

Ishihara plates for colour vision testing

This is a small book of colour 'plates' for colour vision testing (Fig. 2.19). It is useful to test colour vision in suspected optic nerve disease because **colour vision often decreases earlier and more severely than visual acuity in many types of optic nerve disease.** To use the Ishihara colour plates:

- Hold the book at a normal reading distance from the patient.
- Ask the patient to tell you what numbers are on each page, one eye at a time, reading glasses on.
- Count and record the number of correct answers out of the total number of pages with numbers on them, e.g. 'Ishihara 9/15' (9 correct out of 15 number pages).

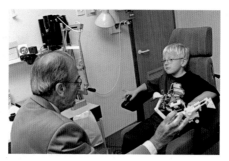

Fig. 2.20 Examining a child.

EXAMINING YOUNG CHILDREN'S EYES

See p. 133 for more details on this. Young children are much more difficult to examine than adults because they:

- Can't tell you what is wrong (the history is from the parents rather than the patient).
- Are unable to read the visual acuity chart.
- Often present with turned eyes (squint/strabismus), which is a much rarer condition in adults.
- Are often uncooperative with the examination.

HISTORY

- Ask about the presenting complaint, e.g. squint: at what age did it appear and how rapid was the onset?
- Specific questions:
  - do the parents think the child can see? (as appropriate for age)
  - are there any symptoms of brain disease? (e.g. headache, vomiting, problems walking?)
  - birth and developmental history
  - was the child premature? (associated with an increased risk of eye problems)
  - did the child experience any developmental delay? (genetic, neurologic or metabolic disease)
  - family history of childhood eye problems? (congenital cataract, retinoblastoma, high refractive error and squint often run in families).

EXAMINATION

- Can the child see with both eyes open? Observe – most children can:
  - keep eye contact with their parents at about 6 weeks of age
  - show interest in bright objects at 2–3 months
  - fix and follow objects with their eyes at 3–4 months
  - can the child see and pick up small objects or sweets?
- Do the two eyes see equally well?
  - repeat the above tests with one eye covered
  - is there an equal objection to covering each eye? (the child won't mind having a blind eye covered).
- Check the child's eye alignment when looking straight ahead – are the eyes looking in the same direction? (See p. 133.)
- Check the child's eye movements (see p. 134).
  - do both eyes move fully in all directions?
  - are there any abnormal repetitive eye movements? (e.g. nystagmus, see p. 165.)
- Is there a normal red reflex with the direct ophthalmoscope? (See p. 30.)
- Check for relative afferent pupillary defect as above.
- Ophthalmoscopy (this is often difficult).

VISUAL LOSS

CROSS-REFERENCES

Visual loss with a red eye: see Chapter 4 The red eye.
Visual loss due to trauma: see Chapter 5 Eye trauma.

OVERVIEW

Every patient with unexplained visual loss requires ophthalmic referral. Most patients with visual loss can be seen routinely, but for a few patients their only chance to recover vision is to have treatment within a few hours of seeing you. Likewise, the cause of visual loss in most patients is eye disease but in a minority of patients the decreased vision is the first sign of a brain tumour. How best then to triage 'blurred vision'?

Visual loss *Critical points*

- **Any patient with unexplained visual loss requires ophthalmic referral.**

- **If visual loss is sudden or rapidly progressive, referral must be *urgent*** (ideally, the patient should be seen the same day).

- **Beware of 'worse than expected' vision:** a level of vision that is worse than would be expected from visible intraocular disease can indicate the presence of optic nerve or brain visual pathway disease.

- **Not all visual loss is caused by eye disease:** the first symptom of orbit or brain tumours and strokes can be blurred vision.

- **Serious eye or brain disease is likely if a patient with blurred vision also has one or more of the following *symptoms*:**
  - unexplained eye pain
  - sensitivity to light (photophobia)
  - distortion of vision (metamorphopsia)
  - flashes of light
  - new-onset floating spots

Continues

Visual loss **Critical points**—cont'd

> - loss of part of the visual field
> - symptoms of temporal arteritis (in patients over 50; see p. 216).

- **Serious eye or brain disease is likely if a patient with blurred vision also has one or more of these *signs*:**
  > - red eye
  > - visual field defect
  > - relative afferent pupil defect (RAPD; see p. 25)
  > - abnormality of the cornea, iris or pupil
  > - loss of the red reflex
  > - optic disc swelling or pallor.

APPROACH TO A PATIENT WITH VISUAL LOSS

ASK

ASK

PRESENTING COMPLAINT

- Is the problem in one or both eyes?
  > - *Caution*: patients with bilateral visual field loss, e.g. from a stroke or brain tumour, might misinterpret the vision problem, believing it to be only in the eye with the more prominent field loss.
- Was the visual loss transient (temporary) or persisting?
- How rapid was the visual loss? Did it occur over:
  > - minutes, e.g. retinal vascular occlusion
  > - days, e.g. retinal detachment
  > - months, e.g. cataract or slowly-progressive optic neuropathy.
- What part of the patient's vision is affected:
  > - just in the centre – suggests macular or some optic nerve diseases
  > - only the left or right side of the visual field – suggests brain visual pathway disease
  > - 'blurred all over' – any cause.

SPECIFIC QUESTIONING

- Pain or photophobia? (these occur in some acute optic neuropathies, migraine, meningitis).
- Distortion of vision? (suggests macular disease).

- 'Flashes', 'floaters' or field loss?:
  - flashes of light: possible retinal detachment
  - new-onset floaters: retinal detachment, diabetic vitreous haemorrhage
  - field loss: retinal, optic nerve or brain visual pathway disease.
- Symptoms of temporal arteritis (in patients over 50, see p. 216)?

PREVIOUS OPHTHALMIC HISTORY

- Does the patient usually wear glasses or contact lenses?
- Previous eye laser or surgery? *Caution*: **patients with visual loss after recent eye surgery require urgent referral.**

PREVIOUS MEDICAL/SURGICAL HISTORY

- Diabetics have an increased risk of serious eye disease.
- Hypertension.

MEDICATIONS

- Any eye drops currently?
- Any tablets that can cause eye toxicity (see Chapter 10)?

FAMILY HISTORY

- Glaucoma, retinal detachment other eye problems?

LOOK FOR

VISUAL ACUITY

See Chapter 2 (How to examine an eye patient) for examination techniques.

VISUAL FIELDS

See Chapter 2 (How to examine an eye patient) for examination techniques. Test to confrontation.

PUPILS

Including the 'swinging torch' test for relative afferent pupillary defect (see p. 25). This is a very important test and should be performed for *all* patients complaining of blurred vision.

LOOK AT THE EYE CAREFULLY WITH A TORCH

- Is it red? (if so, see p. 83).
- Are there abnormalities of the cornea, anterior chamber or iris?

SLIT LAMP EXAMINATION

INTRAOCULAR PRESSURE

Measure with a tonometer (if available).

OPHTHALMOSCOPY (PREFERABLY AFTER USING A DILATING EYE DROP)

- Look for the red reflex. If not present, a dense cataract, vitreous haemorrhage or widespread retinal disease is likely.
- Look at the optic discs. Are they normal, cupped, swollen or pale?
- Look at the retinal vessels, peripheral retina and macula if possible (difficult unless a dilating drop has been used).

TRANSIENT VISUAL LOSS

DIAGNOSTIC FLOWCHART 3.1: TRANSIENT VISUAL LOSS

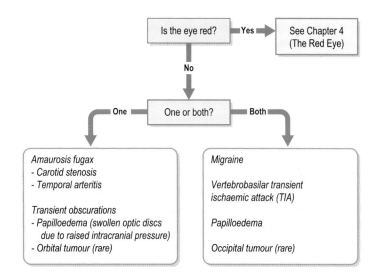

Temporary blurring of vision in one or both eyes is most commonly due to migraine, or transient lack of blood supply to the retina or the brain's visual cortex:

- Retinal ischaemia causes blurring of vision in one eye only.
- Brain ischaemia or migraine causes blurred vision or field loss in both eyes, although the patient might interpret this as being in only one eye. The duration of visual loss and associated symptoms can often suggest the cause.

One eye, severe vision loss, lasts up to an hour: amaurosis fugax

- Usually due to an embolus from a stenosed carotid artery on the same side transiently blocking off the central retinal artery.
- Can also be an early symptom of temporal arteritis.
- **Amaurosis fugax is an important warning sign of impending blindness or stroke, and must not be ignored.**
- Refer to ophthalmologist for full eye examination.
- Urgent (same day) referral if temporal arteritis is suspected; otherwise semi-urgently.

INVESTIGATIONS

- Urgent erythrocyte sedimentation rate (ESR) and C-reactive protein (CRP) if symptoms or signs of temporal arteritis present (both are usually markedly elevated if the patient has temporal arteritis).
- Carotid artery ultrasound, to look for stenosis.
- If no carotid stenosis, investigate the heart for cardiac embolic source.

TREATMENT

- Temporal arteritis: urgent steroid treatment (see p. 217).
- Severe carotid stenosis: refer to vascular surgeon to consider carotid endarterectomy to reduce risk of stroke.
- If no carotid or cardiac source identified: commence long-term, low-dose oral aspirin to try to reduce the risk of permanent eye arterial occlusion or stroke.

One or both eyes, lasts seconds: transient visual obscurations

- These are often associated with papilloedema (swollen optic discs due to raised intracranial pressure, e.g. from a brain tumour).
- Vision loss is very short-lived and might be precipitated by coughing, straining or bending over.
- Any patient reporting these symptoms needs a **careful optic disc examination** and urgent investigation if bilateral optic disc swelling is seen.

Both eyes, lasts minutes to hours, with or without 'sparkling lights' or 'zig-zag lines': occipital visual cortex symptoms

Sparkling blank areas of vision and/or zig-zag lines (scintillating scotomata) are most commonly due to migraine. However, these symptoms can also signify serious brain disease, such as occipital lobe vascular malformation or tumour:

● **Do not attribute these symptoms to migraine unless the patient is under 50, has a definite history of true migraine headaches and has no other neurological symptoms or signs.**

MIGRAINE

● Classically, visual prodrome of scintillating scotomata, blurred vision and/or field loss (both eyes), followed by headache with nausea/vomiting and photophobia.
● However acephalgic migraine can occur (visual symptoms with no headache).
● Normal eye examination and visual field testing after the episode.
● Specific migraine treatments.

VERTEBROBASILAR TRANSIENT ISCHAEMIC ATTACK (TIA)

● Transient homonymous field loss affecting the vision in both eyes (e.g. the patient temporarily loses the right half of the right eye's visual field and the right half of the left eye's visual field because of transient loss of blood supply to the left occipital visual cortex).
● Usually *no* sparkling lights or zig-zag lines.
● Often with transient associated brainstem symptoms (e.g. arm or leg numbness or weakness, problems talking, collapse).
● Normal eye examination and visual fields after the episode.
● Check blood pressure; exclude cardiac embolic source; aspirin (or warfarin if frequent – consult vascular specialist).

OCCIPITAL CORTEX LESION

● Visual cortex tumours or vascular malformations can produce localised seizure activity, which can produce transient homonymous field loss and/or scintillating scotomata.
● In these cases there is often a permanent visual field defect visible on formal visual field testing.
● Any patient with migrainous visual symptoms but no history of migraine, or with other neurological symptoms, needs ophthalmic referral for examination and formal visual field testing.

SUDDEN OR RAPIDLY PROGRESSIVE VISUAL LOSS

DIAGNOSTIC FLOWCHART 3.2: SUDDEN OR RAPIDLY PROGRESSIVE VISUAL LOSS

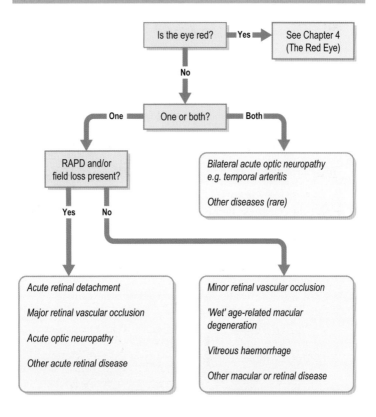

RETINAL VASCULAR OCCLUSIONS

Central retinal vein occlusion (CRVO) (Fig 3.1)

The central retinal vein is occluded by clot, causing retinal haemorrhages and oedema.

SYMPTOMS

- Sudden visual loss in one eye – mild to severe.

SIGNS

- Decreased visual acuity (mild to severe).
- If severe: relative afferent pupillary defect present.
- Widespread retinal haemorrhages, tortuous dilated retinal veins, macular oedema, optic disc swelling, +/– cotton wool spots.

INVESTIGATIONS

Look for risk factors:
- Chronic glaucoma: measure intraocular pressure (IOP), examine the other optic disc.
- Hypertension: check blood pressure.
- Diabetes: check blood glucose level.
- If under age 50: test for blood-clotting disorders.

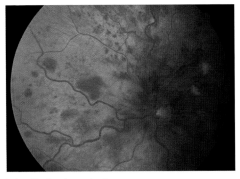

Fig. 3.1 Central retinal vein occlusion.

MANAGEMENT

- Semi-urgent referral.
- Treat underlying cause, if found.
- Pan-retinal photocoagulation (PRP) laser by ophthalmologist if abnormal blood vessels grow in the retina or iris (new vessels in the iris can cause severe painful *rubeotic glaucoma*).

Branch retinal vein occlusion (BRVO) (Fig. 3.2)

A retinal branch vein is occluded (often where it crosses a branch artery, due to hypertension), causing haemorrhage and oedema in the retina it drains.

SYMPTOMS

- Sudden blurring of vision in one eye, and/or sudden loss of part of the visual field.

SIGNS

- Decreased visual acuity.
- Visual field defect.
- Sectoral retinal haemorrhage and oedema, macular oedema, +/− cotton wool spots.

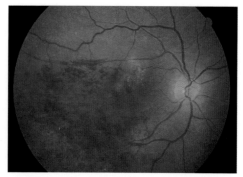

Fig. 3.2 Branch retinal vein occlusion.

INVESTIGATIONS

Look for risk factors:
- Hypertension: check blood pressure.
- Diabetes: check blood glucose level.
- High cholesterol.

MANAGEMENT

- Semi-urgent referral.
- Treat underlying cause, if found.
- Retinal laser by ophthalmologist:
  - if abnormal new retinal vessels grow (they can bleed and cause vitreous haemorrhage)
  - in selected cases, to try to improve poor vision due to macular oedema.

Central retinal artery occlusion (CRAO) (Fig. 3.3)

- The central retinal artery clots off (usually from atherosclerosis) starving the retina of blood.

SYMPTOMS

- Sudden painless loss of all vision in one eye.

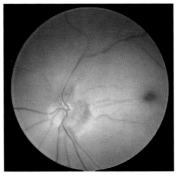

Fig. 3.3 Central retinal artery occlusion.

SIGNS

- Very poor visual acuity (often 'perception of light' only).
- Marked relative afferent pupil defect.
- Retina pale with central macular 'cherry red spot'; poor blood flow through retinal vessels.

INVESTIGATIONS

Look for cause:
- Temporal arteritis (ask about symptoms; see p. 216) and obtain urgent erythrocyte sedimentation rate and C-reactive protein in all cases).
- Hypertension: check blood pressure.
- Diabetes: check blood glucose level.
- High cholesterol.
- A carotid or heart embolic source is uncommon.

MANAGEMENT

- **Immediate urgent referral** (ideally within 1 hour) to ophthalmic emergency centre.
- Occasionally, vision can be restored if an ophthalmologist can lower the intraocular pressure immediately (with medical treatment or by draining aqueous fluid).
- Treat underlying cause, if found.

Branch retinal artery occlusion (BRAO) (Fig. 3.4)

- A branch artery is occluded by an embolus, usually from a stenosed carotid artery.

SYMPTOMS

- Sudden painless loss of a section of visual field in one eye, +/− blurring of central vision.

SIGNS

- Usually decreased visual acuity (sometimes just a visual field defect).
- Sectoral retinal pallor, attenuated branch artery, +/− visible retinal embolus in vessel (these signs can be subtle and are easily overlooked).

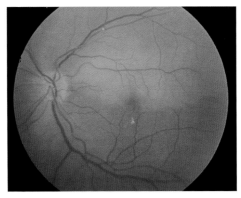

Fig. 3.4 Branch retinal artery occlusion.

INVESTIGATIONS

Look for cause:
- Temporal arteritis (ask about symptoms (see p. 216) and obtain urgent erythrocyte sedimentation rate and C-reactive protein in all cases).
- Carotid stenosis – the most common cause: request carotid ultrasound.
- Heart valve disease: perform a cardiac ultrasound if carotid normal.
- Hypertension: check blood pressure.
- Diabetes: check blood glucose level.
- High cholesterol.

MANAGEMENT

- Semi-urgent referral.
- Treat underlying cause if found.

RETINAL DETACHMENT

- The retina is normally closely adherent to the inside of the eye wall.
- If a tear develops in the retina, vitreous fluid can pass through the tear and underneath the retina, stripping it from the eye wall (*rhegmatogenous* retinal detachment) (Fig. 3.5).

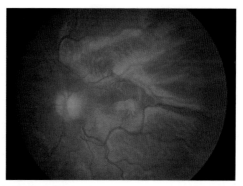

Fig. 3.5 Retinal detachment.

- The detachment usually progresses from a peripheral tear towards the central high-acuity visual area (the macula) – this usually takes hours or days to occur but occasionally can take months.
- Less commonly, the growth of abnormal retinal blood vessels in proliferative diabetic retinopathy pulls the retina off the eye wall (*traction* retinal detachment).

SYMPTOMS

One or more of:
- **Flashing lights** (photopsias) – like lightning or camera flashes.
- **Floating spots** (black or red) of recent onset.
- **Field loss** – like a black or grey curtain slowly coming in from the periphery of one eye, or a blank patch noticed in the vision.
- Blurring of the central vision.

SIGNS

If the macula is still unaffected ('macula-on' detachment), visual acuity may be normal but there might be:
- A visual field defect on confrontation field testing.
- A relative afferent pupillary defect.

Once the macula has detached ('macula-off' detachment), visual acuity is decreased and there is usually a large relative afferent pupil defect and field defect.

SLIT LAMP AFTER DILATING DROPS:

- 'Tobacco dust' (fine brown pigment specks) is often seen in the anterior vitreous behind the lens.

OPHTHALMOSCOPY

- The red reflex might look abnormal in advanced retinal detachment.
- The detached retina looks greyish and wrinkled.
  Caution: **It is very difficult to see a retinal detachment with a direct ophthalmoscope because of its very small field of view. Hence a 'normal' direct ophthalmoscope examination does *not* exclude retinal detachment.**

MANAGEMENT

- **Urgent (same day) ophthalmic referral.**
- Severe vision loss can be prevented if a 'macula on' detachment can be repaired with surgery before the macula is detached.
- If the macula has detached by the time of surgery, there is a poor prognosis for the return of good central vision – the longer the macula has been detached before diagnosis, the worse the visual outcome.

VITREOUS HAEMORRHAGE (Fig. 3.6)

The vitreous cavity lies between the lens anteriorly and the retina posteriorly. Haemorrhage into this cavity can be caused by:

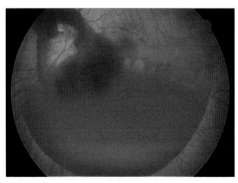

Fig. 3.6 Vitreous haemorrhage.

- Tearing of normal retinal blood vessels, e.g. a retinal tear caused by posterior vitreous detachment (an age change in the vitreous jelly).
- Bleeding of abnormal retinal blood vessels, e.g. in proliferative diabetic retinopathy.
- Blunt or sharp (penetrating) eye trauma.

SYMPTOMS

- Floating blobs or spots if mild or moderate.
- Severe visual loss in one eye if a major haemorrhage.

SIGNS

- Visual acuity normal or reduced.
- Isolated vitreous haemorrhage (without retinal detachment or other retinal disease) does *not* cause a relative afferent pupillary defect.
- If severe: decreased or absent red reflex.

MANAGEMENT

- Urgent referral.

OPHTHALMIC MANAGEMENT

- Treat the underlying cause (e.g. retinal tear or proliferative diabetic retinopathy) with laser or surgery.
- If causing persistent severe visual loss, the vitreous blood can be removed with a vitrectomy operation.

ACUTE OPTIC NEUROPATHIES

An 'optic neuropathy' is any disease that damages the optic nerve.

CAUSES

There are many different causes of sudden-onset optic nerve dysfunction, including:

- Anterior ischaemic optic neuropathy (AION): due to atherosclerosis or temporal arteritis – usually over age 50.
- MS-related optic neuritis: closely related to multiple sclerosis (MS) – usually under age 40.
- Infectious optic neuritis: viral or bacterial – all ages.

- Autoimmune optic neuritis – all ages.
  Overall, the most common types of acute optic neuropathies are MS-related and AION due to atherosclerosis.

TERMINOLOGY

Acute optic neuropathies can affect one or both eyes; they can also affect the anterior or posterior part of the optic nerve:

- **Anterior** optic neuropathies affect the optic nerve head, which causes **optic disc swelling** visible with the ophthalmoscope (Fig. 3.7 left).
- **Posterior** ('retrobulbar') optic neuropathies affect the nerve in the orbit or intracranial cavity, and have a **normal-appearing optic disc** in the early stages (Fig. 3.7 right).

'Optic neuritis' is optic neuropathy in which the optic nerve is inflamed. It is not a specific diagnosis because there are many causes of acute optic nerve inflammation, including infections, autoimmune inflammation and multiple sclerosis.

SYMPTOMS

- Sudden or rapidly progressive loss of vision, one or both eyes.
- Often 'dim' vision or decreased colour vision.
- Sometimes ache or pain behind the eye.
- Symptoms of the underlying disease.

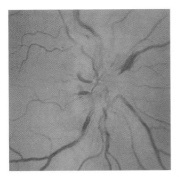 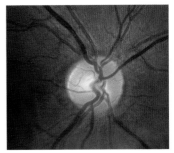

Fig. 3.7 Acute optic neuropathies can have either a swollen (left) or normal (right) optic disc.

- If over age 50, temporal arteritis symptoms might be present – ask specifically about these (see p. 216).
- Symptoms of infections or neurological disease.

SIGNS

- Decreased visual acuity.
- **A relative afferent pupillary defect (RAPD)** is present in unilateral or bilateral asymmetrical optic neuropathies (absent if the optic neuropathy is bilateral and symmetrical).
  - this is a *critical* sign of optic neuropathy of any cause and must be tested for in any patient with visual loss (see p. 25 for details on how to test).
- Visual field: any pattern of visual field loss can occur.
- Usually decreased colour vision in the affected eye(s).
- Ophthalmoscopy: normal or swollen optic disc(s).
  - normal optic disc: in posterior (retrobulbar) optic neuropathies, e.g. in many cases of MS-related optic neuritis and some patients with infectious or inflammatory neuritis
  - swollen optic disc: in anterior optic neuropathies, e.g. anterior ischaemic optic neuropathy (the optic disc undergoes infarction from lack of blood supply).

MANAGEMENT

- **Urgent referral** – with some causes of optic neuropathy specific treatment is possible to reverse damage to the affected eye(s) or, if unilateral, to prevent blindness in the unaffected eye.

MANAGEMENT BY OPHTHALMOLOGIST

- Investigations, if necessary, to determine the underlying cause.

TREATMENT BY OPHTHALMOLOGIST

- Anterior ischaemic optic neuropathy (AION):
  - due to suspected temporal arteritis: urgent steroid treatment, which usually then continues for 1–2 years; temporal artery biopsy to confirm the diagnosis
  - due to atherosclerosis: treat risk factors (e.g. hypertension, diabetes) – some clinicians start long-term aspirin.

- MS-related optic neuritis:
  - complete or almost complete spontaneous recovery of vision usually occurs over a period of days or weeks
  - steroid treatment has no long-term visual or neurological benefit
  - treatments that might reduce the risk of these patients going on to develop other complications of multiple sclerosis are under development.
- Infectious optic neuritis: antibiotic treatment as necessary.
- Autoimmune optic neuritis: steroid treatment often helps.

WET AGE-RELATED MACULAR DEGENERATION

Age-related macular degeneration (ARMD) is a common cause of decreased vision in elderly people. The macula is the central visual area of the retina (the area used for reading and other high-acuity tasks). There are two types of age-related macular degeneration:

- Dry age-related macular degeneration (see p. 67).
- Wet age-related macular degeneration (Fig. 3.8), which is discussed here, is characterized by the sudden distortion or blurring of central vision; this occurs over hours to a few weeks. The blurring is the result of the growth of abnormal new blood vessels under the macula. These vessels then leak fluid or bleed, causing decreased vision.

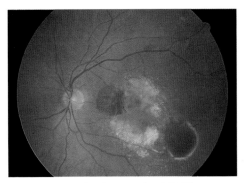

Fig. 3.8 Wet age-related macular degeneration (ARMD).

SYMPTOMS

- Although some patients develop wet age-related macular degeneration in both eyes, it usually affects one eye at a time.
- Acute or subacute blurring of vision in one eye.
- The patient might report:
  - sudden-onset distortion of vision in one eye (metamorphopsia), e.g. straight lines seem curved; the lines of text in a book 'bend'
  - a central blank or blurred patch in the vision (central scotoma), with normal peripheral (side) vision.

SIGNS

- Decreased visual acuity.
- Field testing – the patient might report:
  - a central scotoma on confrontation testing (e.g. when looking at your eye, the patient might say there is a blank patch where your eye is, but that the rest of your face is clear)
  - distortion of the lines or a missing patch on Amsler grid testing (see p. 33).
- Wet age-related macular degeneration does not usually cause a relative afferent pupillary defect, unless it is very extensive.

OPHTHALMOSCOPY

- The affected macula shows oedema (swelling) and / or subretinal haemorrhage and hard exudates.

MANAGEMENT

- Urgent ophthalmic referral.

OPHTHALMIC MANAGEMENT

- Laser treatment can be performed in carefully selected cases. These treatments can, in some cases, prevent or delay the complete loss of central vision but do not usually result in any improvement of vision.
- It is important to ensure that patients with severe bilateral visual loss from age-related macular degeneration are registered for visual impairment assistance and are put in contact with low-vision optical aid specialists and community support groups.

- There is some suggestion that high-dose antioxidant vitamins might slightly decrease the risk of the second eye developing 'wet' changes if one eye has already been affected – research into this is ongoing.

SUDDEN VISUAL LOSS AFTER CATARACT SURGERY

The common causes of sudden decrease of vision in the initial days, weeks or months after cataract (or other intraocular) surgery are:
- Red eye: endophthalmitis.
- White eye: retinal detachment or cystoid macular oedema.
All of these can occur after routine uncomplicated surgery.

MANAGEMENT

- Any patient with a sudden decrease of vision after eye surgery requires **urgent** (same day) ophthalmic referral.

Endophthalmitis

- The onset is usually within days of the surgery (although a rare, mild form occurs after many weeks).
- The patient will report blurred vision, pain and photophobia; the eye is usually red.
- This requires urgent ophthalmic admission for intravitreal antibiotic treatment.
- Visual outcome is often poor but is even worse if the patient is not referred and treated promptly.

Retinal detachment (see p. 51)

Suspect this in any patient who complains of one or more of the following after cataract surgery:
- Sudden decrease of vision.
- Flashes.
- Floaters.
- Field loss (shadow in the peripheral vision).

Cystoid macular oedema

- This is swelling of the macula that occurs a few weeks after cataract surgery.

- People with diabetes are at increased risk.
- Affected patients complain of a blurred spot in the central vision.
- It is very difficult to see macular oedema without a slit lamp retinal lens.
- Treatment involves steroid and non-steroidal anti-inflammatory eye drops in the first instance – most patients improve.

OTHER CAUSES OF SUDDEN VISUAL LOSS

Many hundreds of other eye diseases can cause sudden blurring of vision. A few examples are:

- Retinal infections, e.g. toxoplasma retinitis; cytomegalovirus (CMV) retinitis in AIDS patients.
- Inflammation in the vitreous (posterior uveitis).
- Serous detachment of the macular retina of unknown cause in young adults (central serous retinopathy).

GRADUAL VISUAL LOSS

DIAGNOSTIC FLOWCHART 3.3: GRADUAL VISUAL LOSS

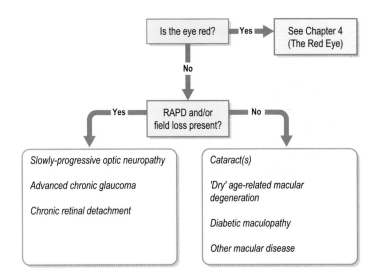

REFRACTIVE ERROR

- Refractive error, or a change in refractive error, is a very common cause of gradual blurring of vision in all ages.
- It is usually a condition that children are born with or develop during childhood.
- We still don't know why this error occurs but it is a mismatch between the amount and type of curvature of the cornea and the length of the eyeball, causing a blurred image to be formed on the retina.

TYPES

MYOPIA ('SHORT SIGHTEDNESS') (Fig. 3.9)
- The eyeball is too long for its focusing power.
- The patient can see near objects clearly, but distance vision is blurred.
- It is corrected with concave ('minus') lenses.

HYPERMETROPIA ('LONG SIGHTEDNESS') (Fig. 3.9)

- The eyeball is too short for its focusing power.
- Younger hypermetropic patients might be able to see clearly without glasses but only with continued effort to focus. If the condition is severe, or in older patients, no objects may be seen clearly, but near objects are more blurred than those in the distance.
- Corrected with convex ('plus') lenses.

ASTIGMATISM

- The cornea is slightly warped, rather than being almost spherical.
- This leads to an image being sharper in one plane than another, e.g. the top horizontal bar of a 'T' on the vision chart might be clear but the lower vertical bar is blurred.
- Corrected with an astigmatic (cylindrical) lens.

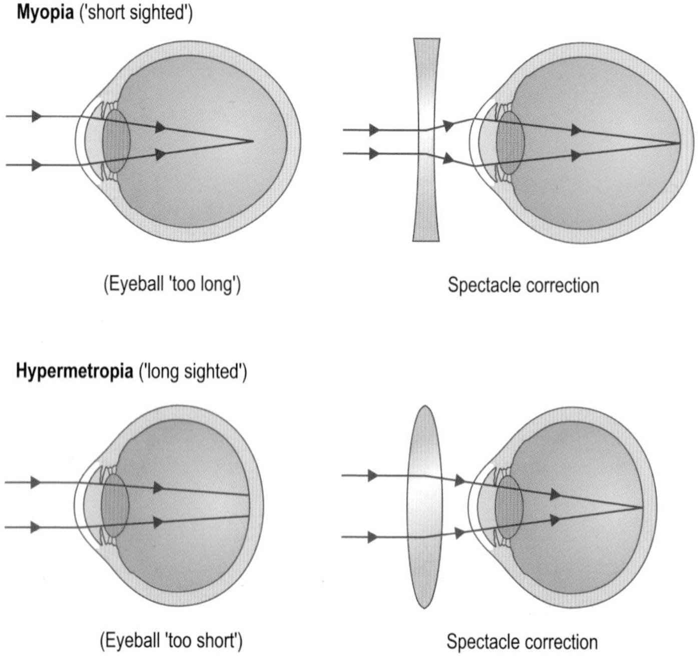

Myopia ('short sighted')

(Eyeball 'too long')   Spectacle correction

Hypermetropia ('long sighted')

(Eyeball 'too short')   Spectacle correction

Fig. 3.9 Types of refractive error.

SYMPTOMS

- Refractive errors in children are often first detected by school vision screening programmes.
- The amount of refractive error can change fairly rapidly until the late teenage years, resulting in frequent (up to yearly) changes in glasses; after that change is usually slow.
- Typical refractive error causes only slowly progressive blurring of vision, which can be fully corrected with a new pair of glasses.
- Rarely, eye diseases (e.g. cataract, intraocular tumours) can cause rapidly changing refractive error.

SIGNS

- The critical sign that refractive error could be causing blurred vision is that visual acuity improves when the patient is tested looking through a pinhole (see p. 23). However, note that acuity in cataract, corneal scars and other conditions can also improve with a pinhole.
- The eye examination should otherwise be completely normal (except in cases of severe myopia, in which there might be secondary retinal degeneration).

MANAGEMENT

- Refer to an optometrist for refraction (measurement of the refractive error) and prescription of glasses.
- If gradual visual loss cannot be fully corrected with glasses, the patient should be referred to an ophthalmologist to examine for other eye disease. This is especially important in children who have been discovered to have poor vision in one or both eyes.
- Contact lenses:
  - these can be considered for adults who don't want to wear glasses or for patients with severe refractive errors (in whom they may provide better vision than glasses)
  - all patients undertaking contact lens wear should be counselled as to the small but serious risk of corneal infections, especially if the lenses are not properly cared for, and should seek urgent help if they develop a red sore eye.

- Refractive surgery:
  - adults who do not wish to wear glasses or contact lenses, and who can afford it, might want to investigate this procedure
  - as with contact lens wear, there is a small but serious risk involved with these procedures.

COMPLICATIONS OF 'PATHOLOGICAL' REFRACTIVE ERRORS

Most refractive error is benign, in that it does not affect the health of the eyeball. However, severe (pathological) myopia or hypermetropia can lead to secondary eye disease:

PATHOLOGICAL (HIGH) MYOPIA

- High risk of retinal detachment.
- Warn the patient to seek urgent ophthalmic assessment if blurred vision, flashes, floaters or field loss ever develop.

PATHOLOGICAL (HIGH) HYPERMETROPIA:

- Increased risk of developing acute glaucoma.
- Warn the patient to see an ophthalmologist urgently if blurred vision, haloes around lights or eye pain develop.

PRESBYOPIA

This condition (uncharitably meaning 'old eye' in Latin) is caused by a decrease in the eye's ability to focus near objects with age. Presbyopia occurs in everyone, whether or not a refractive error has previously been present.

SYMPTOMS

- Onset is usually between the ages of 40 and 50; it occurs earlier in hypermetropes; sometimes later in myopes.
- Vision for distant objects remains clear but reading and other near tasks become increasingly difficult. This can result in books being held further away to read ('My eyes are fine, but my arms are too short!') (Fig. 3.10).

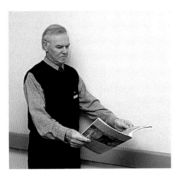 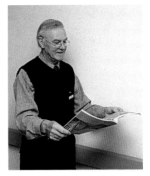

Fig. 3.10 Presbyopia. Left, characteristic problem: 'My arms aren't long enough!'; right, reading glasses solve the problem.

SIGNS

- Normal distance vision.
- Poor near vision.
- Otherwise normal eye examination.

MANAGEMENT

- Refer to optometrist for:
  - reading glasses (if no other refractive error is present, i.e. if glasses were not previously worn)
  - bifocals, varifocals or separate distance and reading glasses (if refractive error is also present, i.e. if glasses were worn previously).

CATARACT

Cataract is a clouding of the normally clear lens of the eye.

CAUSES

- Usually an age-related change, in patients over age 60.
- In younger adults:
  - diabetes (rarely other metabolic diseases)
  - eye trauma
  - intraocular inflammation (e.g. iritis)
  - use of steroid eye drops.

SYMPTOMS

- Gradual blurring of vision in one or both eyes.
- Glare caused by car headlights or sunlight.

SIGNS

- The normally black pupil appears grey or white if cataract is advanced (Fig. 3.11).
- **Cataract, even if very dense, *never* causes a relative afferent pupillary defect (RAPD)**. If this is present, suspect underlying retinal or optic nerve disease.
- Decreased red reflex if advanced.
- Blurred view of the optic disc and retina on ophthalmoscopy.
- Slit lamp appearance: a cataract might have one of the following appearances or be a combination of these:
  - nuclear or nuclear sclerotic cataract: the centre (nucleus) of the lens becomes cloudy but the rest of the lens remains clear; this type of cataract can sometimes cause induced myopia (short-sightedness) and rapid change in the patient's glasses prescription
  - cortical cataract: the outer layers (cortex) of the cataract become opacified but the nucleus remains fairly clear; this type of cataract often causes the patient problems with glare
  - posterior subcapsular cataract: the most posterior layer of the lens becomes opacified; this type of cataract often occurs in patients with a history of intraocular inflammation or steroid eye drop use
  - snowflake cataract: small, white, flake-like opacities develop throughout the lens; although this might the earliest sign of cataract in diabetes, more commonly diabetes causes the common types of nuclear or cortical cataract, but at a younger age than in non-diabetics.

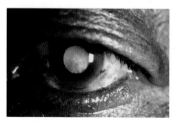 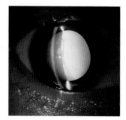

Fig. 3.11 Left, advanced cataract; right, slit lamp view of advanced cataract.

MANAGEMENT

- Routine referral for ophthalmic assessment followed (if required) by cataract extraction and intraocular lens (IOL) implantation.
- Although cataract extraction is a commonly performed and generally very successful procedure, there is a small risk of complications that can cause permanent vision loss. For this reason, the risks of surgery might outweigh the benefit for early cataracts and the patient might instead be observed.

DRY AGE-RELATED MACULAR DEGENERATION

Dry age-related macular degeneration (dry ARMD) (Fig. 3.12) is the most common cause of untreatable visual loss in the developed world. It is the result of a gradual degeneration of the central retinal area (the macula) with age. Many patients only have mild changes and retain reading vision for the rest of their lives; a small number of patients are severely visually handicapped.

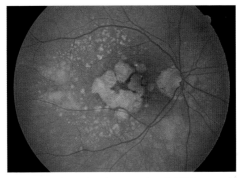

Fig. 3.12 Dry age-related macular degeneration (ARMD).

SYMPTOMS

- Gradual onset of blurred or distorted central vision, usually in both eyes.
- Slow deterioration over many years.
- A minority of patients develop superimposed wet age-related macular degeneration, which causes sudden visual loss (see p. 57).

SIGNS

One or more of these changes at the macula:
- 'Drusen' (yellow dots or blobs – deposits from cell metabolism).
- Retinal pigment epithelial clumping (black spots or patches).
- Areas of 'geographic atrophy' (pale areas).
- *Caution*: **it is difficult to see macular disease with the direct ophthalmoscope,** especially if the pupil has not been dilated; a slit lamp retinal lens is the ideal instrument for macular examination.

MANAGEMENT

- There is no treatment for dry age-related macular degeneration, despite intensive research.
- The patient can be reassured that, even if the loss of central vision is severe, useful peripheral 'navigation' vision is always retained.
- Patients should be cautioned that if they ever develop sudden changes in the vision in either eye, they should present immediately to their ophthalmologist as they might have developed wet changes that could be treatable with laser.
- If vision loss is bilateral and severe it is important to ensure the patient is registered for visual impairment benefits, has the appropriate low-vision optical aids and is in contact with community support groups.

DIABETIC MACULOPATHY

Diabetes can decrease vision in two main ways:
1. Diabetic maculopathy (Fig. 3.13): fluid swelling (waterlogging) of the macula (the central retinal area). This is a common cause of gradual visual loss in diabetics.

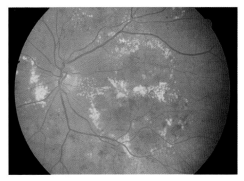

Fig. 3.13 Diabetic maculopathy.

2. Proliferative diabetic retinopathy (abnormal new retinal vessels grow from the retina into the vitreous); this can cause:

   ▶ vitreous haemorrhage (sudden onset of floaters +/– visual loss; see p. 53)
   ▶ traction retinal detachment (gradual or sudden visual loss; see p. 52).

SYMPTOMS

● Patients with early diabetic maculopathy might be asymptomatic and have normal or near-normal visual acuity. Hence routine eye screening of all diabetics is important to detect and treat these cases *before* vision is lost.

● In moderate to advanced cases the patient complains of blurred vision, and sometimes of distorted vision (metamorphopsia).

SIGNS

● It is very difficult to accurately assess diabetic maculopathy without a slit lamp retinal lens examination; direct ophthalmoscope examination can miss early to moderate maculopathy.

● One or more of these in the macular area:

   ▶ microaneurysms (small red dots)
   ▶ small retinal haemorrhages (small red blobs)
   ▶ hard exudates (small yellow deposits)
   ▶ retinal oedema (swelling) – usually visible only on stereoscopic examination with a slit lamp retinal lens.

MANAGEMENT

- **All diabetics require regular eye screening** – at diagnosis and then at regular intervals (usually annually) for the rest of their lives.
- In certain cases of diabetic maculopathy, argon laser treatment to the areas of retinal swelling reduces the risk of future severe visual loss.
- It is important that patients and their doctors understand that the aim of diabetic eye laser treatment is to prevent blindness, not to improve vision – improvement in vision after laser is rare.

SLOWLY PROGRESSIVE OPTIC NEUROPATHIES

An optic neuropathy is any process that damages the optic nerve. Causes include:

- Compression of the optic nerve (by an orbital or brain tumour, or by enlarged extraocular muscles in thyroid eye disease).
- Compression of the optic chiasm (most commonly by a pituitary tumour).
- Infiltration of the optic nerve by tumour or sarcoidosis.
- Toxins, e.g. antituberculosis antibiotics.
- Nutritional deficiency, e.g. vitamin B12 deficiency due to pernicious anaemia or malnutrition.
- Hereditary progressive optic neuropathies.
- Prolonged optic disc swelling of any cause can cause progressive visual loss, e.g. papilloedema due to raised intracranial pressure.

SYMPTOMS

- Gradual decline in vision, one or both eyes.
- Vision might seem 'dimmer' and less colourful in one eye than the other.
- Loss of the central or peripheral visual field might be noticed; patients with pituitary tumours might have trouble driving because of poor peripheral vision.
- Symptoms of the underlying cause, e.g. headaches in some (but not all) patients with tumour; double vision and changed eye appearance in thyroid eye disease.

SIGNS

- Decreased visual acuity and colour vision in the affected eye(s).
- A relative afferent pupillary defect (RAPD) (see p. 25) will be present unless the optic neuropathy is bilateral and symmetrical.
- Visual field defect:
  - any pattern of visual field loss is possible with optic neuropathy of any cause, including central defect (central scotoma) or peripheral defects; no type of field defect is diagnostic of a particular cause
  - if there is chiasmal compression by a pituitary tumour, confrontation testing might reveal a partial or complete bitemporal hemianopia (see p. 212).
- Ophthalmoscopy:
  - the optic disc(s) can look normal or swollen or pale (Fig. 3.14).

MANAGEMENT

- Urgent ophthalmic referral.

OPHTHALMIC MANAGEMENT

- Neuroimaging to exclude a compressive tumour. If such a lesion is found, specific treatment is given.
- Thyroid eye disease causing optic nerve compression: medical or surgical treatment might be necessary to save vision.
- If no compressive lesion found, investigations for other causes.

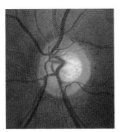 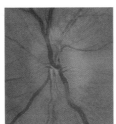 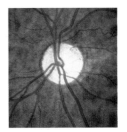

Fig. 3.14 The optic disc in slowly progressive optic neuropathies can be normal (left), swollen (middle) or pale (right).

CHRONIC GLAUCOMA

- Chronic glaucoma is common in the elderly population (it also occurs rarely in children and young adults).
- Abnormally high intraocular pressure is present in most cases, although some patients have normal eye pressure (normal tension glaucoma).
- Progressive damage to the optic nerve head causes characteristic 'cupping' changes from loss of nerve fibres (Fig. 3.15).

SYMPTOMS

- Parts of the peripheral visual field are usually lost long before central visual acuity is damaged.
- **Most patients with chronic glaucoma are asymptomatic and do not notice blurred vision until the disease is very advanced.**

SIGNS

- Normal visual acuity unless advanced.
- The eye looks normal externally (don't confuse this condition with acute glaucoma, which causes sudden-onset painful red eye and blurred vision).

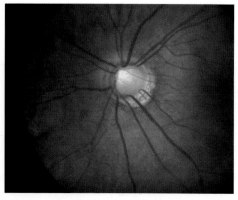

Fig. 3.15 Glaucomatous 'cupping' of the optic disc.

- Visual fields: if advanced, defects might be detectable on confrontation testing; if early or moderate, defects might be visible only on formal visual field testing (e.g. computed perimetry).
- There might be a relative afferent pupillary defect if the glaucoma is advanced and unilateral or asymmetric.
- Intraocular pressure is usually elevated but in up to one-third of chronic glaucoma patients pressure is consistently within the normal range (normal tension glaucoma).
- Pathological cupping of the optic disc is usually visible on ophthalmoscopy:
  - the normal central disc cup (excavated pale area) expands to take up more of the disc than usual, due to nerve fibre death
  - the cup–disc ratio (see p. 32) is usually increased above the normal ratio of 0.5 (i.e. the cup occupies more than half the width of the whole disc).
- There is often also notching (focal loss) of parts of the pink optic disc rim.

MANAGEMENT

- Early detection by screening.
- **Everyone over the age of 40 should have a glaucoma screening test by their optometrist every 2 years** (screening might need to begin earlier if there is a close relative with glaucoma, as this is a known risk factor).
- Central visual acuity can be preserved if patients can be detected by routine screening and treated *before* the disease becomes advanced (although the lost peripheral vision cannot be recovered).
- Routine ophthalmic referral if early glaucoma suspected; semi-urgent referral if advanced optic disc changes and/or severely elevated intraocular pressure.

OPHTHALMIC MANAGEMENT

- Regular, life-long follow-up with monitoring of intraocular pressure, disc appearance and formal visual field testing.
- Intraocular pressure-lowering treatment with eye drops in the first instance.
- If this fails to control the disease progression, pressure-lowering laser treatment (trabeculoplasty) or surgery (trabeculectomy) might be necessary.

GRADUAL VISUAL LOSS AFTER CATARACT SURGERY

The most common causes of gradual decrease in vision months or years after cataract surgery are:
- posterior capsular fibrosis
- other unrelated eye disease, e.g. dry age-related macular degeneration.

Posterior capsular fibrosis (Fig. 3.16)

- This is caused by a slow opacification of the posterior capsule, part of the fine capsular bag from which the cataract is extracted and into which the intraocular lens is inserted.
- Fibrosis occurs in up to one-third of routine cataract surgery patients.

SYMPTOMS

- Gradual decrease in vision and/or increasing glare, months or years after cataract extraction.

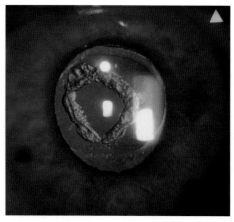

Fig. 3.16 Hole in opacified posterior capsule following YAG laser.

SIGNS

- With the slit lamp (ideally with dilating drops), the fibrosis can be seen as a fine grey/white layer of scar tissue behind the intraocular lens.

MANAGEMENT

- Routine ophthalmic referral, for consideration of YAG laser capsulotomy (a hole is created in the scarred posterior capsule to allow clearer vision).

CHRONIC RETINAL DETACHMENT

- Retinal detachment usually presents either as acute blurred vision or with flashes, floaters and/or acute visual field loss.
- However, in some cases patients report a gradual decrease of the vision in one eye, or a slowly increasing field defect, and are found on examination to have a detachment.

OTHER CAUSES OF GRADUAL VISUAL LOSS

There are hundreds of other causes of gradual vision loss in one or both eyes, for example:

- Toxic maculopathies, e.g. from drug treatment with hydroxychloroquine, thioridizine or tamoxifen.
- Eye tumours such as choroidal malignant melanoma.

THE YOUNG CHILD WITH POOR VISION

CAUSES

- Congenital cataracts.
- Intraocular retinoblastoma.
- Congenital abnormalities of the retina, optic nerve or brain visual system.
- Optic nerve or chiasm tumours.

PRESENTATION

Young children with decreased vision may present with one or more of:

- A turned eye: 'squint' or strabismus (Fig. 3.17):
  - blind eyes in children tend to turn
  - any child with a squint should be suspected of having poor vision until proven otherwise
  - the condition causing poor vision might be serious, e.g. intraocular retinoblastoma or optic nerve tumour.
- Nystagmus (constantly moving eyes):
  - poor vision in both eyes from birth, or with onset in the first few months of life, will cause nystagmus
  - every child with nystagmus has the nystagmus as a result of (not a cause of) bilateral poor vision, until proven otherwise.
- Parents feel the child is slow-developing, e.g. the child does not recognise parents' faces or does not smile.
- The child appears clumsy or runs into objects.
- Specific symptoms, e.g. a child with congenital glaucoma or albinism might be photophobic (discomfort from bright lights).

EXAMINATION

For more information on examining young children's eyes, see Chapter 6.

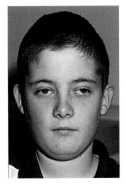

Fig. 3.17 A child with strabismus. The left eye is turned out.

MANAGEMENT

- Any child with suspected poor vision requires prompt ophthalmic referral.
- In many cases, specific treatment is possible to improve vision, e.g. surgery for congenital cataracts.

THE RED EYE

CROSS-REFERENCE

Red eye due to trauma: see Chapter 5 Eye trauma.

OVERVIEW

Many of your patients who present with red eye will have common, benign conditions that you can treat yourself. However, some will have acute, sight-threatening diseases in which even a few hours delay in referral will result in permanent loss of vision. How can you tell who to worry about?

Fortunately, a few questions, visual acuity testing and examination of the eye with a torch (and magnification if you have it) are all that is usually required to triage the serious from the non-serious. As always, if there is any doubt, **refer**.

The red eye *Critical points*

- **All cases of red eye of unknown cause with decreased vision, pain or photophobia require urgent (same-day) referral to an ophthalmologist or ophthalmic emergency department.** Do not prescribe any treatment for these patients before referral – this wastes time and can interfere with investigations.

- **Do not call every red eye 'conjunctivitis'!** There are many other causes of red eye, many of them serious and requiring urgent treatment by an ophthalmologist.

- **The only time you should prescribe antibiotic drops or ointment is for bacterial conjunctivitis:** *two* red eyes, *pus-like* discharge, *normal* vision, *no* pain or photophobia. Red eye(s) of other causes will either resolve with no treatment (e.g. viral conjunctivitis), require a different treatment (e.g. allergic conjunctivitis), or require urgent referral (e.g. iritis or infectious corneal ulcer).

- **Never prescribe steroid or antibiotic–steroid eye drops** unless asked to by an ophthalmologist – serious damage to the eye can occur. *Continues*

The red eye *Critical points*—cont'd

- **A newborn baby with red eyes** and eye discharge has sight- and life-threatening infection (ophthalmia neonatorum; see p. 105) until proven otherwise, and requires urgent ophthalmic review.

APPROACH TO A PATIENT WITH RED EYE(S)

ASK ABOUT

- A history of trauma or foreign body hitting the eye (see Chapter 5 Eye trauma).
- **Blurred vision, pain or sensitivity to light** (photophobia) that you can't explain after a careful examination (i.e. not due to a corneal abrasion or foreign body). **These are all serious symptoms – refer urgently.**
- Haloes around lights as well as blurred vision and pain (acute glaucoma).
- Itch (allergic conjunctivitis).
- Recent viral upper respiratory infection (viral conjunctivitis).
- History of eye disease or operation:
  - red eye with blurred vision in the past could be iritis, dendritic ulcer, marginal keratitis
  - red eye after eye surgery – suspect endophthalmitis: refer urgently.
- Contact lens wearer:
  - be wary of corneal infections – refer early.

LOOK FOR

ONE OR TWO EYES AFFECTED?

TEST VISION: NORMAL OR DECREASED?

TEST PUPILS

- Abnormal pupil size, shape or poor reaction to light in a red eye is a sign of serious eye disease, e.g. acute glaucoma or iritis.

ASK

LOOK FOR

LOOK FOR

LOOK AT THE EYE
Use light and magnification:

- How red is the eye and where is the redness? There are three patterns of redness:
1. *Ciliary injection:* redness greatest in a ring around the peripheral cornea, often seen in iritis, acute glaucoma, and other serious causes of red eye. However, this pattern of redness should not be relied on for diagnosis.
2. *Conjunctival injection:* diffuse redness of the whole conjunctiva, often seen in conjunctivitis.
3. *Subconjunctival haemorrhage:* a thin continuous layer of bright red blood overlying the white sclera.

- Is there any discharge?
  - yellow pus-like discharge: in both eyes in bacterial conjunctivitis; in one eye in severe corneal ulcer
  - clear, watery discharge; in viral or chronic infectious conjunctivitis.
- Examine the cornea: is it clear, or is there a foreign body or ulcer?
- Examine the anterior chamber (the space between the clear cornea and coloured iris): is there a fluid level of pus (hypopyon) or blood (hyphaema) (Fig. 4.1)?
- Anterior chamber 'depth' is very difficult to assess without a slit lamp but sometimes in acute glaucoma the iris can be seen to be almost pressed up against the back of the cornea ('shallow' anterior chamber).

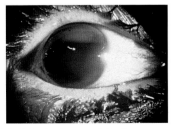 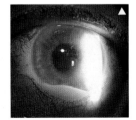

Fig. 4.1 Left, hyphaema; right, hypopyon.

- Stain the cornea with fluorescein and look with a blue light:
  - uniform diffuse yellow glow is normal (except in acute chemical burn or severe infection, when it can signify a total epithelial defect)
  - corneal ulcers or abrasions appear as a well-demarcated area of bright yellow staining (an epithelial defect)
  - if the substance of the cornea (stroma) under this is crystal clear, the diagnosis could be traumatic corneal abrasion, viral dendritic ulcer or other conditions mainly affecting the epithelium (the surface layer of the cornea)
  - if the substance of the cornea under this is cloudy or white, the diagnosis could be a bacterial, viral or fungal infectious corneal ulcer.
- Evert the eyelids (top and bottom):
  - is there a foreign body under the upper eyelid?
  - are there lumps on the inside surface of the eyelids?
  - papillae (fine pink 'cobblestones'): in both eyes in bacterial or allergic conjunctivitis
  - follicles (small grey 'rice grains'): in one or both eyes in viral conjunctivitis.

OPHTHALMOSCOPY
- Difficult if the patient is photophobic.
- It is best not to dilate the pupil with drops in acute red eye with decreased vision before referral.

CHECK THE INTRAOCULAR PRESSURE
- Every patient with one red eye and unexplained pain or decreased vision must have an urgent eye pressure check to exclude acute glaucoma.
- Normal intraocular pressure is less than 21 mm of mercury (mmHg).
- Acute glaucoma is likely if the pressure is very high (usually more than 40 mmHg).

ONE RED EYE, DECREASED VISION

DIAGNOSTIC FLOWCHART 4.1: ONE RED EYE, DECREASED VISION

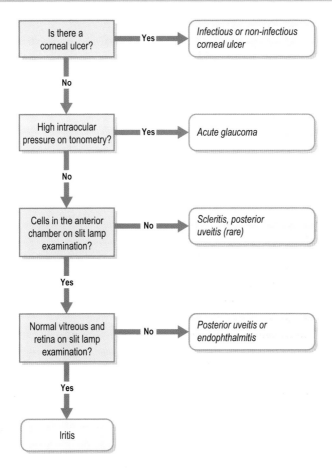

The following serious causes of red eye are usually unilateral, although they can occasionally affect both eyes together.

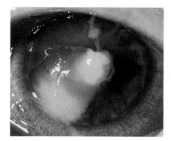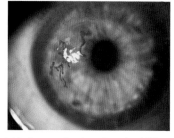

Fig. 4.2 Left, bacterial corneal ulcer; right: herpes simplex virus dendritic corneal ulcer.

INFECTIOUS CORNEAL ULCER

- Causes include bacteria (Fig. 4.2, left), fungi, viruses (including herpes simplex virus (Fig. 4.2, right), the cause of dendritic ulcer).
- **Contact lens wearers** are at greatly increased risk of corneal infections.

SYMPTOMS

- Pain, foreign body sensation, blurred vision, photophobia.

SIGNS

- Mild to severe redness.
- (Usually) decreased visual acuity.
- Red eye (often 'ciliary injection': redness maximal around the edge of the cornea).
- Viewing the cornea with white light:
  - viral dendritic ulcer: there might be no obvious abnormality
  - bacterial or fungal ulcer: white or yellow area in the normally clear cornea (corneal infiltrate).
- Fluorescein plus blue light: an area of corneal epithelial defect (staining yellow) is seen:
  - usually in a branching (dendritic) pattern if herpes simplex virus is the cause
  - other causes: irregular area of staining overlying the corneal infiltrate.
- Hypopyon (pus) in the anterior chamber in severe cases.

MANAGEMENT

- **Urgent ophthalmic referral.**
- **Do not start any treatment before referral** – the use of topical antibiotics before ophthalmic assessment can cause delay in referral and makes culturing the causative agent of the infection difficult.

OPHTHALMIC MANAGEMENT

- Dendritic ulcer due to herpes simplex: topical aciclovir ointment.
- Possible bacterial or fungal keratitis: take corneal culture sample then commence frequent broad-spectrum antibiotic drops and follow closely – the patient might require admission to hospital if severe.

NON-INFECTIOUS CORNEAL ULCER

CAUSES

- Autoimmune disease, e.g. rheumatoid arthritis.
- Exposure keratopathy, e.g. in patients with seventh nerve palsy (facial palsy) who can't close the eyelids on one side.
- Severe dry eye.
- Atopic keratitis (in a patient with severe facial eczema).
- Neurotrophic keratopathy (ulcer due to numb eye, e.g. from trigeminal nerve disease).
- Contact lens related non-infectious ulcer.

SYMPTOMS

- Foreign body sensation, pain (except in neurotrophic), blurred vision.

SIGNS

- Mild to severe redness.
- Can appear identical to a corneal abrasion (see p. 116) or an infectious corneal ulcer (see above).
- Signs of underlying cause, e.g. poor eyelid closure, severe dry eye, numb cornea, severe atopic skin and eyelid disease.

MANAGEMENT

- Urgent ophthalmic referral.
- Treat specific cause, e.g. frequent lubricants +/– lid surgery for seventh nerve palsy.

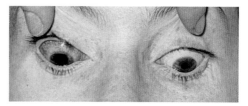

Fig. 4.3 Acute glaucoma.

ACUTE GLAUCOMA (Fig. 4.3)

- This is a sudden severe rise in intraocular pressure (IOP).
- Usually due to occlusion of the 'angle' of the anterior chamber (where aqueous fluid is normally drained): 'acute angle-closure glaucoma'.
- If unrelieved for more than a few hours, very high intraocular pressure can cause permanent visual loss.

SYMPTOMS

- Sudden-onset aching eye pain, which is often severe and can be accompanied by nausea and vomiting.
- Blurred vision +/– rainbow-like 'haloes' around lights.

SIGNS

- Red eye (can be mild or severe).
- Decreased visual acuity (mild or severe).
- Cloudy cornea (corneal oedema) if severe.
- Anterior chamber depth (the distance between the cornea and iris) might be shallow.
- Pupil often mid-dilated and not reactive to light.
- **Very high intraocular pressure on testing with tonometer:**
  - usually over 40 mmHg (normal eye pressure is less than 22 mmHg)
  - *all patients with unexplained red eye and pain or blurred vision must have their intraocular pressure measured urgently to exclude acute glaucoma.*

MANAGEMENT

● **Urgent ophthalmic referral.**

OPHTHALMIC MANAGEMENT

● Urgent medical treatment to decrease intraocular pressure.
● Then YAG laser iridotomy:
   ◗ in acute angle closure the normal path of aqueous fluid from the ciliary body where it is produced to the drainage angle is blocked where the iris presses against the lens
   ◗ laser holes shot through the peripheral iris produce an alternative route for the aqueous flow and intraocular pressure often returns to normal.

IRITIS (ANTERIOR UVEITIS) (Fig. 4.4)

● Inflammation in the iris and anterior chamber of the eye, with no abnormalities anywhere else in the eye (normal vitreous and retina).
● Usually autoimmune and of unknown cause; sometimes due to infections or specific autoimmune diseases.
● Usually unilateral, however, it can be bilateral.

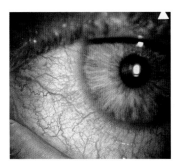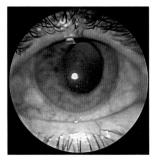

Fig. 4.4 Iritis. Left, circumciliary injection; right, keratic precipitates (KPs).

SYMPTOMS

- Usually young or middle-aged patients.
- Blurred vision, photophobia (bright lights hurt the eye), pain if severe.
- Sometimes a history of autoimmune disease associated with iritis, e.g. ankylosing spondylitis, inflammatory bowel disease.

SIGNS

- Red eye(s) (may be mild initially).
- Decreased vision (only mild initially).
- Usually clear cornea.
- If severe, the pupil might be small or irregular and constrict poorly to light.
- Hypopyon (pus in anterior chamber) if severe.
- **Slit lamp:**
  - *iritis can't be diagnosed without a slit lamp microscope examination*
  - turn the slit lamp light to maximum, adjust the beam so it is short and narrow, and angle the beam through the anterior chamber at about 45 degrees; the room lights should be off
  - cells (fine, moving, white specks) and flare (the normally invisible light beam looks like a car headlight through fog) are seen in the anterior chamber
  - keratic precipitates (KPs; clumps of inflammatory cells) might be seen on the inner aspect of the cornea.
- Ophthalmoscopy:
  - often difficult due to photophobia
  - normal vitreous and retina (unless also posterior uveitis).

MANAGEMENT

- **Urgent (same-day) ophthalmic referral.**
- *All patients with an unexplained red eye and pain, photophobia or blurred vision must have a careful slit lamp examination of the anterior chamber to exclude iritis.*

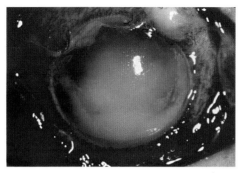

Fig. 4.5 Endophthalmitis.

OPHTHALMIC MANAGEMENT

- Exclude inflammation at the back of the eye (which can spill forwards and mimic iritis).
- Intensive topical steroids plus dilating drops initially; sometimes systemic immunosuppression required.
- Test for underlying infective or autoimmune condition if atypical, refractory, bilateral or recurrent.

ENDOPHTHALMITIS

Endophthalmitis (Fig. 4.5) is a severe inflammation extending throughout the interior of the eyeball, involving both the aqueous and vitreous compartments.

CAUSES

- Infection after eye surgery.
- Infection after penetrating eye injury or traumatic eyeball rupture.
- Infection spreading to one or both eyes through the blood stream, e.g. from infected heart valves in endocarditis or contaminated needles in intravenous drug users.

SYMPTOMS

- Blurred vision, 'floaters', aching pain in the eye, photophobia.

SIGNS

- Decreased visual acuity.
- Signs of iritis.
- (Sometimes) hypopyon (pus in the anterior chamber).
- A relative afferent pupillary defect (RAPD) might be present if the retina has been damaged or detached.
- Decreased red reflex.
- Eyelid swelling.

MANAGEMENT

- Urgent ophthalmic referral and admission.
- If postsurgical or post-traumatic: vitreous biopsy and intravitreal and topical antibiotics.

RED EYE(S), NORMAL VISION

For traumatic causes of red eye with normal vision, see Chapter 5 Eye trauma.

DIAGNOSTIC FLOWCHART 4.2: ONE RED EYE, NORMAL VISION

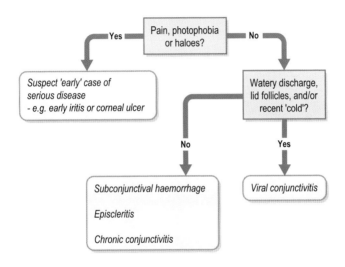

DIAGNOSTIC FLOWCHART 4.3: TWO RED EYES, NORMAL VISION

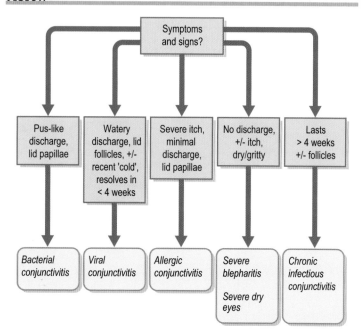

BACTERIAL CONJUNCTIVITIS (Fig 4.6)

SYMPTOMS

- Might be briefly unilateral, but usually becomes bilateral.
- Red, sticky, gritty eyes with pus-like discharge (but no pain or photophobia).
- Family members or co-workers are often affected (it is very contagious).

SIGNS

- Two red eyes.
- Yellow, pus-like discharge.
- Diffuse ('conjunctival') redness of the ocular surface.

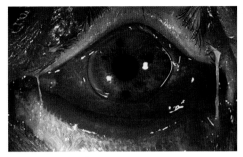

Fig. 4.6 Bacterial conjunctivitis.

- Lid eversion: papillae (cobblestone-like, small, pink lumps).
- Normal visual acuity.
- Normal corneas, anterior chambers and pupils.

INVESTIGATIONS

- None required initially – bacterial swabs are not routinely required unless there is no response to treatment within a week or atypical features are present.

MANAGEMENT

- Topical antibiotic drops to both eyes, 2-hourly while awake for 2 days then 4 times a day for a week.
- Warn patients that they are contagious for as long as the eyes are red.
- **Refer if:**
  - decreased vision, pain or photophobia at any stage
  - not better in 2 weeks.

VIRAL CONJUNCTIVITIS (Fig. 4.7)

SYMPTOMS

- **One or two eyes** red, watery, gritty.
- (Often) symptoms of a current or recent viral upper respiratory infection.

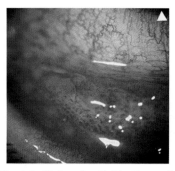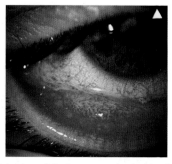

Fig. 4.7 Viral conjunctivitis; the greyish 'grains of rice' spots on the inside of the lower lid are follicles.

SIGNS

- One or two red eyes – diffuse redness of the ocular surface ('conjunctival injection').
- Clear, watery discharge (no pus).
- Lid eversion: follicles (small grey lumps that look like tiny grains of rice).
- Normal visual acuity.
- Normal corneas, anterior chambers and pupils.
- (Sometimes) enlargement of the pre-auricular and/or cervical lymph nodes; other signs of viral infection.

MANAGEMENT

- **Antibiotic eye drops have no effect on viral conjunctivitis.**
- **Topical steroid treatment is not necessary in most cases and should never be started, except by an ophthalmologist.**

TELL THE PATIENT

- They have an eye infection with a virus similar to that which causes the 'common cold'.
- Antibiotics will not help and they will get better by themselves.
- It can sometimes take up to 3 weeks for the redness to resolve.
- They are highly contagious while the eye is red, and should avoid contact with other people – they should avoid touching their eyes,

wash their hands frequently and use a separate towel to other household members. (Make sure you don't get it yourself, or give it to your next patient! Wash your hands carefully.)

- If the redness clears and their vision remains normal, they do not need to see you again.
- **They need to be seen urgently by an ophthalmologist if:**
  - vision decreases at any stage
  - the eye becomes painful (rather than just irritated)
  - they are no better in 2 weeks.

ALLERGIC CONJUNCTIVITIS

Allergic conjunctivitis (Fig. 4.8) can occur:

- As a chronic or recurrent problem in allergic people (asthma, hayfever, eczema).
- As an acute contact allergy to eye drops, contact lens cleaning solution, cosmetics, plant material etc.

SYMPTOMS

- **Itch** is the predominant symptom.
- This can be seasonal, e.g. worse in spring (due to increased pollen).

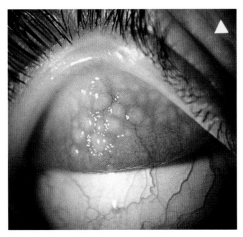

Fig. 4.8 Allergic conjunctivitis: large papillae under the everted upper lid.

- Intermittent or chronic eye redness.
- There might be some mucous or watery discharge but this is not usually copious.

SIGNS

- Mild redness might be present or the eyes might not appear inflamed at all.
- Lid eversion: papillae (fine, pink, 'cobblestone-like' lumps), especially under the upper lids.
- Normal visual acuity and cornea.

MANAGEMENT

- Avoid the allergen if possible, if a contact allergy.
- Try treatment with topical mast cell inhibitor, e.g. cromoglycate or lodoxamide drops t.d.s. in both eyes for a 2-month trial (it can take several weeks to achieve a full effect). If successful, this can be safely continued long term (or seasonally as necessary).
- If there is also a component of dry eye, 'artificial tears' can be used when needed.
- Routine ophthalmic referral if distressing symptoms persist.
- **Steroid eye drops should only ever be commenced under ophthalmic supervision**, and for as short a time as possible. Long-term use can give patients (who are often young) cataracts or irreversible visual loss from glaucoma.

INFECTIOUS CHRONIC CONJUNCTIVITIS

'Chronic' conjunctival infections might initially look like bacterial or viral conjunctivitis. However, they last more than 4 weeks. Causes include:
- Atypical bacterial conjunctivitis.
- Chlamydial inclusion conjunctivitis.
- Trachoma.

Atypical bacterial conjunctivitis

- Unusual or resistant organisms requiring specific antibiotic drops.
- Perform conjunctival swab for bacterial culture.
- Also test for chlamydial inclusion conjunctivitis, or (if dry rural area) trachoma.

Chlamydial inclusion conjunctivitis

- A sexually transmitted eye disease of young adults.

SYMPTOMS AND SIGNS

- Persistent follicular conjunctivitis (resembling viral conjunctivitis) in one or both eyes for more than 4 weeks.
- If chronic, conjunctival scarring and peripheral corneal inflammation can occur.
- The patients might also have symptoms of chlamydial urethritis.

INVESTIGATION

- Special conjunctival swab test for chlamydia (a 'standard' bacterial swab culture will not detect this organism).

TREATMENT

- 2 weeks oral doxycycline (avoid if pregnant or breast-feeding).
- Test for other sexually transmitted diseases.
- Refer sexual partners for testing.

Trachoma

- An endemic infectious disease of dry rural areas associated with poverty and poor hygiene, spread by flies and direct contact.
- A major cause of preventable blindness (400 million people affected world-wide).
- Children are often acutely infected, with the infection then becoming chronic; acute infection can resemble viral conjunctivitis.
- Chronic sight-threatening complications of the eye surface can occur.

INVESTIGATION

- Special conjunctival swab test (if available).

TREATMENT

- Ideally, refer to ophthalmologist; however, this might be difficult due to lack of availability, poverty and remote location.
- Suspected acute cases are treated with a single dose of oral azithromycin or longer courses of other antibiotics.
- Public health measures are vital to decrease endemic disease in affected communities.

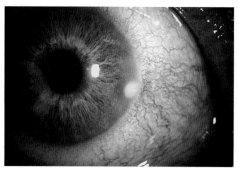

Fig. 4.9 Marginal keratitis.

MARGINAL KERATITIS (Fig. 4.9)

- This is usually a mild, non-infectious ulceration of the peripheral cornea, caused by a peripheral corneal reaction to chronic eyelid inflammation (chronic blepharitis).
- Rarely, severe sight-threatening marginal keratitis can occur due to infections or autoimmune disease (e.g. in rheumatoid arthritis).

SYMPTOMS

- Sudden increase in eye irritation and foreign body sensation, usually on a background of chronic gritty/irritated eyes.
- No significant pain, photophobia or blurred vision (unless severe).

SIGNS

- Mild localised eye redness (often only surrounding the involved sector of the cornea).
- Normal visual acuity (suspect serious cause if not).
- Fluorescein with blue light: small peripheral corneal ulceration with underlying mild corneal haze.
- Often 'bridging' fine blood vessels from the conjunctiva to the ulcer.

MANAGEMENT

- Urgent ophthalmic referral to exclude infectious and autoimmune causes.

OPHTHALMIC MANAGEMENT

- If marginal keratitis secondary to blepharitis:
    - treat with topical antibiotics plus steroids, under close ophthalmic supervision until healed.
- Treat chronic blepharitis with hot lid compresses and lid scrubs twice a day long-term to try to prevent recurrence (see p. 202).

RECURRENT CORNEAL EROSION

This is a small, non-infectious, spontaneous corneal epithelial defect that appears weeks to years after an initial traumatic corneal abrasion. This occurs because the corneal epithelium that regrows over a traumatic defect might not be as tightly adherent as it was before the original injury, and peels off again with minimal or no trauma.

SYMPTOMS

- Sudden onset of foreign body sensation (can be severe) – often on waking in the morning.

SIGNS

- Usually normal (or near-normal) visual acuity.
- Eye redness may be minimal or absent.
- The cornea looks normal with a white torchlight.
- Fluorescein plus blue light: small area of yellow fluorescein staining (can be anywhere on the cornea) – the underlying cornea is clear (not white or cloudy as in bacterial ulcer).

MANAGEMENT

- Urgent ophthalmic referral to exclude corneal ulceration of other causes (e.g. dendritic ulcer).

OPHTHALMIC TREATMENT

- The acute ulceration usually heals within a few days with eye patching and/or lubricants.
- However, erosions often recur and can become problematic for the patient.
- Prevention involves frequent use of lubricants (including lubricant ointment at night, to decrease the chance of recurrent erosion in the morning).

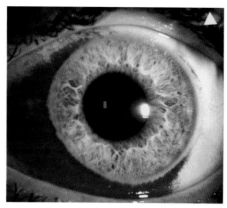

Fig. 4.10 Subconjunctival haemorrhage.

SPONTANEOUS SUBCONJUNCTIVAL HAEMORRHAGE (Fig. 4.10)

This is the spontaneous appearance of bright red blood between the white sclera and the overlying thin transparent conjunctiva. This often looks very dramatic and is worrisome for the patient. It is usually benign, although occasionally it might be the presenting sign of systemic disease.

CAUSES

- (Usually) no cause can be identified.
- Eye rubbing.
- Severe coughing or straining.
- Rarely, severe hypertension or blood clotting disorders.

SYMPTOMS

- Often noticed incidentally by the patient or relatives.
- Sometimes mild foreign body sensation at onset.
- No blurred vision, pain or photophobia.

SIGNS

- Diffuse area of bright red blood under the conjunctiva of one eye (this looks different to most 'red eyes', which are dilation of the fine conjunctival and scleral blood vessels).
- Normal visual acuity.
- Eye examination otherwise normal.

INVESTIGATIONS

- Check the blood pressure in all patients.
- If recurrent or severe, or if a history of other unexplained bruising or bleeding, check full blood count and blood coagulation studies.

MANAGEMENT

- Investigate as above if indicated.
- Reassure patients as to the benign nature of the condition and tell them it could take 2 weeks or more for the redness to resolve.
- Refer if recurrent, persistent or severe.

EPISCLERITIS (Fig. 4.11)

This is a mild, self-limited inflammation of the episclera (a fine connective tissue layer between the white sclera and the overlying clear conjunctiva).

SYMPTOMS

- Mild eye irritation and redness.
- No significant itch or discharge.
- No significant pain or photophobia.

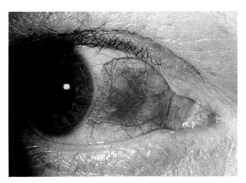

Fig. 4.11 Episcleritis.

- Redness of the eye – usually mild, usually sectoral (sometimes diffuse).
- Normal visual acuity.
- Otherwise normal ocular examination.

- Mild: no treatment – almost all resolve spontaneously.
- Discomfort and/or redness persisting for more than 2 weeks: ophthalmic referral for consideration of treatment with topical steroids or non-steroidal agents.
- **Do not start steroid treatment yourself, unless under instruction from an ophthalmologist.**

SCLERITIS (Fig. 4.12)

- An inflammation of the white sclera itself.
- It is usually **painful** (compared with episcleritis, which is uncomfortable rather than painful).
- As opposed to episcleritis (which usually occurs in otherwise healthy patients), patients with scleritis often have serious underlying systemic vasculitis.

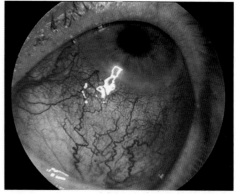

Fig. 4.12 Scleritis.

SYMPTOMS

- Mild to severe aching eye pain (often wakes the patient at night).
- Vision normal early on, but may later become severely reduced due to ocular complications.

SIGNS

- Diffuse or sectoral redness of the eye.
- The eye is often tender to touch.
- Vision normal or decreased.
- There might also be:
  - peripheral corneal ulceration
  - signs of intraocular inflammation.

MANAGEMENT

- Urgent ophthalmic referral for investigation and treatment.
- Ophthalmic treatment may involve oral immunosuppressive agents.

CONTACT LENS PROBLEMS

Contact lens wearers are prone to both minor and serious corneal diseases.

- **A contact lens wearer with a red eye plus pain, photophobia, or decreased vision has an infectious corneal ulcer until proven otherwise.**

Conditions contact wearers have an increased risk of include:

Corneal ulcers (Fig. 4.13)

- **Refer urgently to an ophthalmologist.**
- Non-infectious ulcers:
  - from severe overwear, poorly-fitting lenses, poor lens hygiene, or traumatic lens insertion or removal
  - if small and peripheral, vision might be normal and the patient complains of foreign body sensation rather than pain.
- Infectious corneal ulcer:
  - often more painful than non-infectious ulcers
  - affect central or peripheral cornea
  - due to bacteria, or unusual organisms (e.g. fungi or *Acanthamoeba*)
  - if early, vision might be normal.

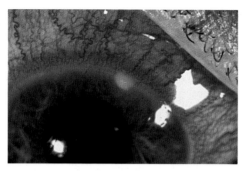

Fig. 4.13 Contact-lens-related peripheral corneal ulcer.

Other problems

Refer to the optometrist or ophthalmologist who prescribed the lenses if the patient describes:

- Chronic irritation: poor fit of lenses or dirty lenses.
- Chronic itch: allergy to the lens cleaning solution or lens material.
- Contact lens overwear: this can cause persistent irritation, vascularisation and scarring of the peripheral cornea.
- Sleeping in lenses: this is usually not serious if it occurs occasionally but it can sometimes cause hypoxic corneal inflammation.
- Difficulty removing the lenses: can cause extensive corneal abrasions.

OTHER CAUSES

There are many other less common causes of persistent red eye(s) with normal vision, including:

- Pterygium or inflamed conjunctival tumour.
- Low-flow carotid-cavernous fistula.
- Autoimmune chronic conjunctivitis, e.g. ocular pemphigoid.

RED EYE IN A NEONATE

OPHTHALMIA NEONATORUM

This is a general term for eye infections in new-born babies (within the first 2 weeks of life). These are often due to sexually transmitted diseases passed during birth from the mother to the baby. Causative organisms include:

- **Gonorrhoea** – this is very serious and can cause:
  - bilateral severe infectious corneal ulcers resulting in perforation of both corneas and bilateral blindness
  - bloodstream spread with fatal meningitis or encephalitis without urgent intravenous antibiotic treatment.
- **Chlamydia** – often less severe than gonorrhoea, but still serious:
  - discharge can be purulent or watery
  - sometimes associated with a serious chlamydial lung infection
  - treat with intravenous antibiotics.
- **Herpes simplex virus** – usually watery discharge; can be associated with severe systemic infection and requires intravenous antiviral treatment.
- **Other** 'common' bacteria – these are less serious than the above.

New-born babies also often have congenital nasolacrimal duct obstruction, which can cause chronic watering and sticky discharge from one or both eyes. This does not cause red eye, red eyelids or severe eye discharge and hence should not be confused with ophthalmia neonatorum.

RED EYE IN A CHILD

- Red eyes in children are caused by similar diseases as in adults (with the exception of acute angle closure glaucoma, which is rare).
- Examination can be difficult because of poor cooperation and difficulty assessing critical signs such as visual acuity in preverbal children.
- Serious disease, such as iritis and endophthalmitis, can still occur in children.
- For this reason, **any child with a red eye in whom visual acuity cannot be measured requires urgent ophthalmic referral for further examination.** In some cases this might require examination under general anaesthetic to exclude serious ocular disease.

EYE TRAUMA

CHAPTER CONTENTS

OVERVIEW

Anyone who has worked in an emergency department on a Friday night knows that 'black eyes' are common, and usually benign. However, some patients presenting with blunt trauma have sight-threatening complications, such as eyeball rupture or retinal detachment; sharp trauma or a high-speed foreign body striking the eye can also cause loss of vision. Detecting these serious eye injuries *early* is important. Sometimes, if the injury is missed during the initial trauma assessment, the opportunity to save vision or to save the eye is lost.

Eye 'trauma' can also occur with minimal force, for example a corneal abrasion from a fingernail, or a corneal foreign body that has blown into the eye. These injuries can still be very painful for the patient and it is important to treat them correctly.

Eye trauma *Critical points*

- **If a high-velocity foreign body has hit the eye, consider that it is *in* the eye until proven otherwise** (by X-ray or CT scan, and careful ophthalmic examination).

- **If you suspect your patient has a possible penetrating eye injury, an urgent telephone consultation with an ophthalmologist is required to plan emergency transfer and surgery.** Keep the patient nil by mouth, place a hard shield (not a soft patch) over the eye, and give antiemetics and analgesia as required.

- **Any patient with head or facial trauma (including a 'black eye') should have a basic eye examination** to exclude serious eye injuries. Every patient with a 'black eye' has serious underlying eye trauma until proven otherwise.

- **Alkali and acid burns** to the eyes are potentially sight-threatening and require urgent thorough eye irrigation (water or saline) for 30 minutes, followed by urgent ophthalmic opinion.

DIAGNOSTIC FLOWCHART 5.1: EYE TRAUMA

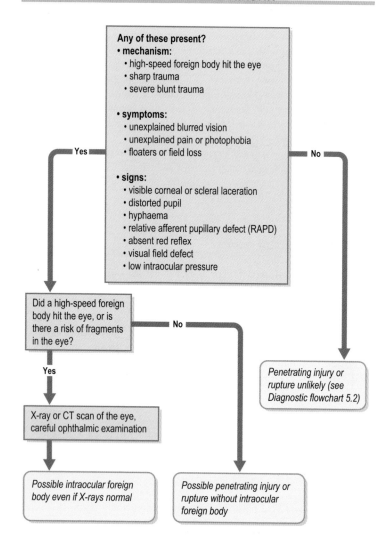

Any of these present?
- **mechanism:**
  - high-speed foreign body hit the eye
  - sharp trauma
  - severe blunt trauma

- **symptoms:**
  - unexplained blurred vision
  - unexplained pain or photophobia
  - floaters or field loss

- **signs:**
  - visible corneal or scleral laceration
  - distorted pupil
  - hyphaema
  - relative afferent pupillary defect (RAPD)
  - absent red reflex
  - visual field defect
  - low intraocular pressure

Yes

No

Did a high-speed foreign body hit the eye, or is there a risk of fragments in the eye?

No

Yes

X-ray or CT scan of the eye, careful ophthalmic examination

Penetrating injury or rupture unlikely (see Diagnostic flowchart 5.2)

Possible intraocular foreign body even if X-rays normal

Possible penetrating injury or rupture without intraocular foreign body

DIAGNOSTIC FLOWCHART 5.2: PENETRATING INJURY OR RUPTURE UNLIKELY

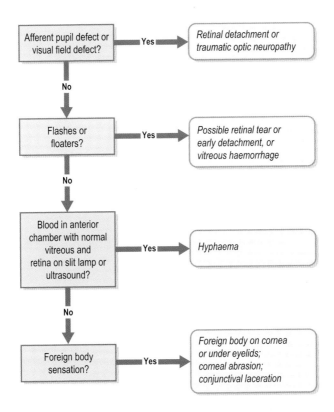

See also:
- Chemical burns (p. 125)
- Eyelid lacerations (p. 120)
- Decreased vision after blunt trauma (p. 123)
- Double vision after blunt trauma (p. 123)
- Unequal pupils after blunt trauma (p. 124).

APPROACH TO A PATIENT WITH EYE TRAUMA

In each case, consider:
- What other injuries are present? Life-threatening injuries must always be looked for and take precedence.
- What is the nature of the injury? Was it:
  - foreign body hit the eye
  - sharp trauma
  - blunt trauma
  - a burn (chemical or thermal).
- Exclude acute sight-threatening injury, e.g. eyeball rupture or perforation.
- **Eyelids 'swollen shut' from bruising:**
  - by drying the skin and prying the eyelids open with your fingers or cotton buds, the patient's vision can almost always be assessed and a view of the eye can be obtained
  - if this is impossible, the orbit should be imaged on CT scan or ultrasound to determine whether the eyeball is ruptured.
- **If the patient is unconscious:**
  - pupils might be small and poorly reactive due to narcotics; this will make assessment for a relative afferent pupil defect (RAPD) and ophthalmoscopy very difficult (but still try, with the room lights down)
  - *dilated pupil(s)* in an unconscious patient can signify a dangerous increase in intracranial pressure causing compressive third nerve palsy, and may require urgent neuroimaging. For this reason, do *not* use dilating drops in patients on 'neuro observations'.
- **If the patient is drunk or uncooperative:** do the best you can and then also re-examine later.

ASK

PRESENTING COMPLAINT
- Nature of injury?
- **Did the patient feel something hit the eye?**
  - *if history of a high-speed metal fragment hitting the eye, suspect intraocular foreign body and order an urgent X-ray.*
- Blunt trauma: what was the patient hit with?
- Chemical burn: what was the chemical? (and find out the pH – but start irrigation first)

ASK

SPECIFIC QUESTIONING

- Is the vision blurred? (penetrating eye injury, ruptured globe, hyphaema, vitreous haemorrhage, retinal detachment, traumatic optic neuropathy, retinal 'bruising' (commotio)).
- Pain? (bruising, corneal abrasion or laceration, ruptured globe, hyphaema, orbit wall fracture).
- Foreign body sensation? (foreign body on the cornea or conjunctiva or under the upper lid; or corneal or conjunctival abrasion or laceration).
- Double vision? (nerve palsy due to intracranial or orbit trauma, or orbital wall fracture).
- Flashes, floaters, field loss? (retinal tear or detachment, or vitreous haemorrhage).

PREVIOUS OPHTHALMIC HISTORY

- Previous eye operation? (increases the chance of eyeball rupture with blunt trauma).
- Contact lens wearer? (is the contact lens still in the eye? If so, remove if the patient is unconscious or going to be admitted to hospital).

LOOK FOR

LOOK FOR

VISUAL ACUITY

- Distance visual acuity chart with distance glasses on (or pinhole if usual glasses not available).
- If patient bed-bound: can they read the small or large print of a newspaper or magazine? (test each eye in turn).

FIELD TESTING

- Visual field defect suggests retinal detachment or traumatic optic neuropathy.

RELATIVE AFFERENT PUPILLARY DEFECT (RAPD)

- If relative afferent pupil defect is present in one eye, retinal detachment or traumatic optic neuropathy is likely (see p. 25 for how to test).

LOOK FOR

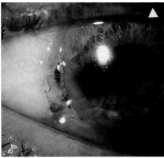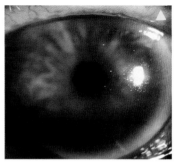

Fig. 5.1 Left, iris distortion and prolapse due to penetrating injury; right, hyphaema.

LOOK AT THE EYE CAREFULLY WITH A TORCH

Use magnification, if available, and a slit lamp if you have one and the patient is mobile. Signs of possible serious eye disease are:

- Cloudy cornea.
- Blood in the anterior chamber (between the cornea and the iris) – hyphaema (Fig. 5.1, right).
- Irregular-shaped or unreactive pupil.
  - in penetrating eye injury or ruptured globe the pupil might be 'tear-drop' shaped, pointing to the site of rupture, due to iris prolapsing out of the rupture site (Fig 5.1, left; don't mistake this for a foreign body and try and remove it!).
- If none of the above, and the patient reports foreign body sensation, always evert ('flip') the upper lid to look for a foreign body under the lid.

OPHTHALMOSCOPY

- Is the red reflex present and is there a clear view of the optic disc? If not, possible vitreous haemorrhage from ruptured globe, or retinal detachment.
- Are the optic discs normal? Look especially for bilateral optic nerve head swelling in severe head injury (this indicates high intracranial pressure).

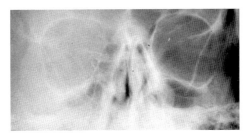

Fig. 5.2 Intraocular foreign body on X-ray.

ORDER RADIOLOGY

- **X-ray the eye if the patient says a small foreign body has hit the eye with speed, even if your examination is normal.**
  - it is possible to have a small intraocular foreign body (Fig. 5.2) with a very subtle penetration wound, normal or near-normal vision, and a comfortable eye!
  - be particularly suspicious if the patient was hammering metal and reported that something flew up and hit the eye; this often causes a penetrating injury
  - patients often report that something has hit the eye while they were grinding metal; this more often causes a corneal or conjunctival foreign body than a penetrating injury.
- **X-ray the orbit** for possible orbital wall fracture if one or more of:
  - double vision
  - bony tenderness around the eye
  - decreased sensation on the cheek or upper teeth
  - you can feel air under the skin around the eye ('surgical crepitus').
- **CT scan or ultrasound** the eye if the eyelids are completely shut and can't be opened, to exclude eyeball rupture.

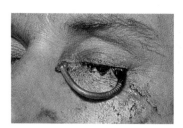 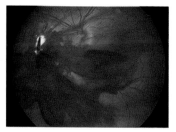

Fig. 5.3 Left, penetrating injury with nail; right, ophthalmoscopic view of posterior eye wall perforation in 'through and through' penetrating injury.

FOREIGN BODY HIT THE EYE

Small foreign bodies include pieces of metal (common when the patient's work includes grinding metal or welding), or small pieces of vegetable matter or soil. If a patient reports that a small foreign body 'blew' or fell into the eye, a penetrating eye injury is highly unlikely. However, if the history is that the foreign body hit the eye at speed or with force (e.g. a metal splinter from hammering metal, or glass from a smashed windscreen), a penetrating eye injury +/− intraocular foreign body must be excluded as a matter of urgency.

Larger foreign bodies can cause a spectrum of injury, from corneal abrasion to ruptured globe.

PENETRATING EYE INJURY ± INTRAOCULAR FOREIGN BODY

- In penetrating injury, an object perforates full-thickness through the cornea or sclera (Fig. 5.3).
- In some cases, a foreign body is retained within the eye (intraocular foreign body).
- Penetrating eye injury is a serious threat to vision because:
  - the original injury can damage intraocular structures, causing cataract, retinal detachment or vitreous haemorrhage
  - in many cases, **infection** is introduced, which progresses rapidly to endophthalmitis (infection throughout the interior of the eye)
  - this can result in loss of all vision, or even the eye itself
  - the risk of infection is increased if an intraocular foreign body is present.
- The sooner the injury is diagnosed and repaired with urgent surgery, the better the visual prognosis.

SYMPTOMS

- Occult penetrating injury can be present despite minimal pain or visual disturbance – suspect based on the mechanism of injury.
- Symptoms can include one or more of:
  - blurred vision
  - flashes, floaters and/or field loss (from vitreous haemorrhage or retinal detachment)
  - foreign body sensation
  - pain
  - photophobia.

SIGNS

One or more of:
- Decreased visual acuity (usually, although occasionally this is normal early after the injury).
- Red eye (usually).
- If a relative afferent pupil defect (RAPD) or field loss is present, retinal or optic nerve damage has occurred.
- Visible corneal or scleral wound.
- Prolapse of pigmented iris or ciliary tissue through the wound.
- Distorted pupil: the pupil may be drawn into a 'teardrop' shape, with the 'point' pointing to the site of the corneal or scleral laceration (due to prolapse of the iris through the wound).
- Hyphaema (blood in the anterior chamber).
- Cataract (a lens that has been penetrated or lacerated will rapidly become cloudy or white).
- Vitreous haemorrhage – if severe may cause loss of the red reflex.
- Low intraocular pressure (IOP) if measured (but in general *avoid* measuring intraocular pressure if you suspect a penetrating injury).

MANAGEMENT

- **Urgent referral.**
- Immediate management by the diagnosing doctor:
  - **telephone** the eye surgeon on call, so they can prepare to receive the patient
  - **keep the patient nil by mouth** (he or she will be having emergency general anaesthetic soon after arrival at hospital)
  - **cover the eye with a hard shield** (commercial or improvised, e.g. cut the bottom off a disposable drinking cup) – **do not use an eye pad** – to prevent any pressure on the eye (Fig. 11.1, bottom right)

⬧ **do not put any eye drops on the eye**
⬧ give **pain relief** if needed
⬧ **treat vomiting** with anti-emetics if required (vomiting increases pressure in the eye).

● If emergency transfer will take some time, the receiving surgeon might request an initial dose of intravenous antibiotics to cover against infection.

OPHTHALMIC MANAGEMENT

● Look for intraocular foreign body by examination and imaging.
● Urgent microsurgical repair of the entry wound in the eye wall.
● Repair of secondary ocular damage (e.g. vitreous haemorrhage or retinal detachment) either during initial surgery or as a second later procedure.
● Treat infection if present or suspected.

CORNEAL ABRASION (TRAUMATIC EPITHELIAL DEFECT)
(Fig. 5.4)

● A traumatic defect in the corneal epithelium (thin superficial layer of the cornea).
● This can occur with even minor trauma, e.g. a scrape with a finger or difficult removal of a contact lens.

SYMPTOMS

● Foreign body sensation ('Something is in my eye').
● Pain (this can be severe).
● Photophobia.
● There might be blurring of vision if central.

SIGNS

● Red eye.
● Visual acuity usually normal or mildly decreased.
● There is a defect in the corneal epithelium (this is much more easily visible with fluorescein drops and a blue light).
● The underlying and surrounding corneal substance is *clear* (i.e. no white or yellow infiltrate suggestive of infection).
● The eye examination is otherwise normal.

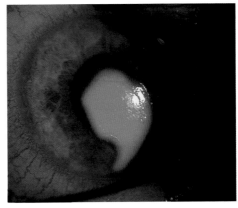

Fig. 5.4 A corneal abrasion staining yellow–green with fluorescein dye, viewed with a blue torch light.

MANAGEMENT

- Refer urgently if vision is significantly decreased or you are concerned there could be other eye injuries.
- If vision is good and you are confident that the abrasion is the only injury, put antibiotic ointment on the eye and apply a firm double eye pad (see p. 226 for the technique).
- Review the patient within 24 hours:
  - if the abrasion is healing, re-apply ointment and pad and review in 24 hours
  - even large abrasions should be completely healed within 3 days
  - if the defect is unchanged or worse, refer urgently for ophthalmic assessment.

CORNEAL FOREIGN BODY

Note: many patients present with corneal foreign bodies without a history of 'getting something in the eye'.

SYMPTOMS

- Foreign body sensation.
- Pain, photophobia – usually mild to moderate; if severe, infection is possible and the patient should be referred.

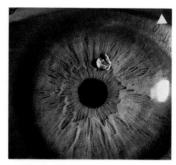

Fig. 5.5 Corneal metal foreign body.

SIGNS

- Visual acuity normal (if a small peripheral foreign body) or mildly decreased (central foreign body or secondary infection).
- Foreign body on the cornea (Fig. 5.5) (if this is small it might be visible only with magnification).
- Rarely, signs of superimposed infectious ulcer (white or yellow corneal infiltrate).

MANAGEMENT

- Remove the foreign body if possible (see p. 228 for the technique).
- Antibiotic ointment and double eye pad; review within 24 hours.
- **Refer urgently to an eye emergency department if:**
  - you are concerned the foreign body could be **full-thickness** through the cornea
  - you are suspicious of **infection** (white or yellow area surrounding the foreign body; severe blurring of vision, severe pain or photophobia)
  - the foreign body is **central** in the cornea (i.e. the size of the scar from removal will be visually important) or deep
  - the foreign body (or rust ring around it) **cannot be removed completely** ('going back and having another try tomorrow' usually doesn't help).
- Corneal foreign bodies in young children often require referral for removal under a brief general anaesthetic.

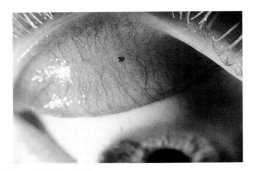

Fig. 5.6 Subtarsal foreign body.

FOREIGN BODY UNDER THE UPPER EYELID: SUBTARSAL FOREIGN BODY (Fig. 5.6)

Note: many patients have subtarsal foreign bodies without a history of getting anything in the eye. If a patient complains of foreign body sensation and no cause is found, 'flip' (evert) the upper eyelid (see p. 27 for the technique).

SYMPTOMS

- Scratchy/gritty foreign body sensation.

SIGNS

- Red eye (usually mild).
- There are sometimes vertical scratches on the upper half of the cornea if a foreign body is under the upper lid (best seen with fluorescein drops and a blue light).
- Foreign body seen on the inner surface of the upper eyelid after lid eversion.
- Otherwise normal examination.

MANAGEMENT

- Once a foreign body is found it can usually be wiped off the inner eyelid surface with a cotton bud.

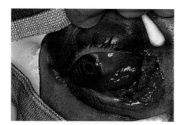 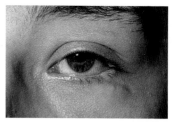

Fig. 5.7 Left, severe lower eyelid laceration; right, following surgical repair.

SHARP TRAUMA

Common causes of sharp trauma are motor vehicle accidents (broken windscreen glass impacting the face) and fights (broken bottles or knives).

CORNEAL OR SCLERAL LACERATION

- Symptoms, signs and management are the same as for penetrating eye injury.

EYELID LACERATION (Fig. 5.7)

The important steps in eyelid laceration are:
1. Exclude other serious injuries, e.g. brain injury.
2. Exclude underlying damage to the eyeball, e.g. corneal or scleral laceration.
3. Exclude damage to the lacrimal drainage system – if the laceration is medial (near the nose), the lacrimal canaliculus may be lacerated and require special repair.
4. Repair the eyelid (Fig. 5.7, right). Ideally, this should be performed by an ophthalmic or plastic surgeon, to avoid long-term functional and cosmetic problems.

BLUNT TRAUMA

RUPTURED EYEBALL

- The sclera splits due to severe blunt force.
- The risk of this is increased if the patient has previously had eye surgery (the old wound can split open).
- Symptoms, signs and management are as for penetrating eye injury.
- Rupture can sometimes occur at the back of the eyeball, which can be more difficult to detect; poor vision, relative afferent pupil defect, loss of the red reflex and a 'soft' eye with low intraocular pressure are clues.

HYPHAEMA

Hyphaema (see Fig. 5.1, right) is blood in the anterior chamber between the clear cornea and the coloured iris.

SYMPTOMS

- Blurred vision.
- If pain is severe, intraocular pressure might be raised.

SIGNS

- Decreased visual acuity.
- The blood fluid level might be visible without magnification ('macroscopic' hyphaema) or the red cells in the anterior chamber might be visible only with the slit lamp ('microscopic' hyphaema).
- No relative afferent pupil defect, unless there is retinal or optic nerve disease.

MANAGEMENT

- **Urgent ophthalmic referral to:**
  - exclude other eye injuries – with slit lamp examination or (if blood is obscuring the view of the retina) ultrasound imaging
  - measure intraocular pressure – secondary acute glaucoma presents the greatest risk to vision from hyphaema (the other sight-threatening complication is permanent corneal blood staining).

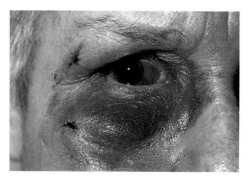

Fig. 5.8 Black eye.

- Bed rest to decrease the chance of re-bleeding.
- Young children need to be admitted to hospital for enforced bed rest and close observation.
- Older children and adults, if reliable and living close to the hospital, can be reviewed frequently as outpatients unless complications occur.
- Monitor and treat the intraocular pressure while the eye reabsorbs the anterior chamber blood.

'BLACK EYE' (PERIORBITAL ECCHYMOSIS)

A 'black eye' is the result of bruising of the skin around the eye (Fig. 5.8). It is not serious or sight-threatening by itself, but it **might conceal other, more serious eye injuries.**

ASSESSMENT

1. **Exclude other serious injuries,** including brain injury.
2. **Exclude underlying eye injury** (e.g. ruptured globe or hyphaema) with a full eye examination:
   - if the eyelid bruising and swelling is severe, the lids may need to be prised open with your fingers or cotton buds to allow eye examination, or at least to determine if the eye can see
   - *if the lids are unable to be opened at all, ultrasound or CT imaging of the eyeball and orbit should be undertaken* to exclude an underlying rupture of the eyeball.

3. **Exclude orbital fracture:** X-ray or CT orbit if any of these are present:
   - double vision or restricted eye movements
   - decreased skin sensation under the eye, or the patient reports numb upper molar teeth (possible infraorbital nerve damage from fracture)
   - proptosis (eyeball pushed forwards)
   - air under the eyelid skin ('surgical crepitus').

- If normal vision, normal ocular examination and no sign of orbital fracture, the patient should be reviewed in 1 week for re-examination.
- The bruising often takes 2 weeks or longer to resolve.
- The patient should also be warned to return immediately at any stage in the future if blurred vision, double vision or symptoms of retinal detachment (flashes, floaters, field loss) occur.
- If an orbital fracture is found on X-ray or CT, this requires semi-urgent ophthalmic referral to assess whether surgical repair is required.

DECREASED VISION AFTER BLUNT TRAUMA

This requires **urgent ophthalmic assessment**. Possible causes (from front to back) are:
- Eyeball rupture.
- Cornea – abrasion.
- Anterior chamber – hyphaema.
- Lens – traumatic dislocation or cataract.
- Vitreous – haemorrhage.
- Retina – bruising ('commotio') or retinal detachment.
- Optic nerve – traumatic optic neuropathy.
- Brain – visual pathway bruising or compression by haematoma.

DOUBLE VISION AFTER BLUNT EYE TRAUMA

See p. 140 for how to assess double vision. Possible causes:
- Orbital +/− extraocular muscle bruising or bleeding, with or without fracture (most commonly).
- Orbital fracture with entrapment of an extraocular muscle.
  - orbital floor 'blowout' fractures can trap the inferior rectus muscle; this causes restriction of both elevation and, to a lesser extent, depression of the eye and requires semi-urgent surgery to free the muscle.

- Cranial nerve palsy (third, fourth or sixth nerve) – due to severe closed head injury, or compression by expanding intracranial haematoma.

ABNORMAL PUPILS AFTER BLUNT TRAUMA

Conscious patient

See p. 157.

Unconscious or drowsy patient

It is often difficult to tell the cause of unilateral or bilateral dilated pupils in an emergency room or intensive care setting. Consider **one or two large pupils** in a patient who is drowsy or unconscious (or recently 'knocked out') as being due to an expanding intracranial haemorrhage until proven otherwise – **perform urgent brain imaging.**

ONE LARGE PUPIL THAT CONSTRICTS POORLY TO LIGHT

- Raised intracranial pressure (causing third nerve palsy):
  - high intracranial pressure from an expanding intracranial haemorrhage can cause pressure on one or both third (oculomotor) nerves, causing dilated pupil(s).
- Traumatic mydriasis:
  - blunt trauma to the iris constrictor muscle, from a direct blow to the eye.
- Dilating drop in one eye.
- Brainstem damage.

TWO LARGE PUPILS THAT CONSTRICT POORLY TO LIGHT

- Raised intracranial pressure (causing bilateral third nerve palsies).
- Traumatic mydriasis (although this is more commonly unilateral).
- Brainstem damage.
- Dilating drops in both eyes.

ONE SMALL PUPIL THAT DILATES POORLY IN THE DARK (RARE)

- The other pupil is abnormally large (from the above causes) plus narcotics.
- Horner's syndrome from neck or head trauma (possible internal carotid artery dissection).
- Brainstem damage.

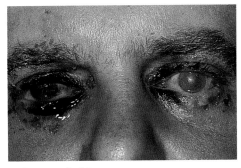

Fig. 5.9 Bilateral severe alkali burn.

TWO SMALL PUPILS THAT DILATE POORLY IN THE DARK (COMMON)

- Usually narcotics (medicinal or illegal).
- Brainstem damage.

BURNS TO THE EYE

CHEMICAL BURN

- These range from mild irritation (e.g. shampoo in the eye) to severe sight-threatening injuries.
- Alkali burns (Fig. 5.9) tend to be more severe than acid burns (except strong acids).

SYMPTOMS

- Pain, blurred vision, foreign body sensation, photophobia.

SIGNS

- Red eye (the exception being that very severe alkali burns can present with an eye that is 'white' due to total loss of the conjunctival blood vessels).
- Signs of severe burn:
  - decreased visual acuity
  - cloudy cornea
  - epithelial defect with fluorescein (might be 100% defect).

FIRST AID MANAGEMENT (BY THE PATIENT, GENERAL PRACTITIONER OR EMERGENCY DOCTOR)

- Do not delay irrigation to examine the eye – irrigate then examine.
- Immediate copious eye irrigation under running water (or saline) for 30 minutes.
- If the patient is in severe pain, apply local anaesthetic drops to allow the eye to be opened for irrigation.
- While irrigating:
  - evert the upper and lower lids to allow full eye surface irrigation
  - remove any particles of chemical matter with a cotton bud if seen.
- Do *not* use pH strips – these just delay (or unnecessarily prolong) irrigation.
- 'Antidote chemicals' are not required (and might increase the damage).
- **Urgent ophthalmic referral.**

OPHTHALMIC MANAGEMENT

- Finish irrigation (if previously inadequate).
- Examine for damage.
- Specific treatments are necessary (as an inpatient) for severe burns.

THERMAL BURN

- Corneal thermal burns can occur after facial exposure to flame or explosion.
- Injuries can consist of:
  - corneal ulceration
  - corneal stromal opacification due to thermal injury.

MANAGEMENT

- Urgent referral to hospital general emergency department.
- Exclude life-threatening respiratory burns.
- Urgent ophthalmic consultation.
- Supportive care to heal the ocular surface (e.g. lubricants, skin grafts to burnt eyelids, or temporary tarsorrhaphy to cover the cornea).

WELDING 'FLASH'

- This can occur when a person is welding without proper eye protection.
- It is an ultraviolet light burn of the corneal surface ('sunburn of the cornea').
- Welding flash rarely causes permanent damage, but can be extremely painful.
- Symptoms are often delayed in onset by 4–8 hours after the exposure (hence sufferers often present to the emergency department at night).

SYMPTOMS

- Usually both eyes.
- Blurred vision, foreign body sensation, pain, photophobia (often severe).

SIGNS

- Red eye(s).
- Visual acuity might be mildly or moderately reduced.
- The corneal stroma is clear.
- Corneal examination (magnifier or slit lamp) with fluorescein drops plus blue light: widespread pinpoints of yellow staining in the corneal epithelium.

MANAGEMENT

- Supportive care until the epithelium heals itself:
  - dilating eye drops reduce the painful photophobia, e.g. cyclopentolate 1%, one drop in each eye stat
  - antibiotic ointment plus firm eye pressure patch (both eyes might need to be patched for comfort if severe)
  - pain-relief tablets as required (do not give local anaesthetic drops to take home, as this can delay healing).
- Can be managed as an outpatient unless pain is very severe.
- Review in 24 hours, at which stage the patient is usually much better.

TURNED EYE/DOUBLE VISION

CHAPTER CONTENTS

TURNED EYE IN CHILDREN

OVERVIEW

A 6-month old child brought to you with an inward-turned eye most likely has idiopathic infantile ('congenital') esotropia. There is a small chance, however, that the child actually has a brain tumour that has caused a sixth nerve palsy, or that the eye has turned because it is blind from a malignant intraocular retinoblastoma. Hence **every child with a 'turned eye' (strabismus or 'squint') requires prompt ophthalmic referral.**

The second important reason for early referral of childhood squints is that if an eye is turned for even a few weeks early in life, or a few months in later childhood, the visual area of the developing brain develops fewer connections with the 'turned' eye than with the 'straight' eye. This results in **amblyopia** (often called 'lazy eye'). In amblyopia, the eyeball itself is normal; it is the connections in the visual cortex that are poorly formed. Amblyopia can cause permanent blindness of the turned eye if it is not detected and treated early.

Unlike adults with new-onset squint, children with early-onset squints who are old enough to talk **do not complain of double vision:** this is because the young brain learns to 'ignore' the turned eye.

'Turned eye' in children Critical points

- **A child of any age with strabismus ('turned eye') has a sight- or life-threatening condition until proven otherwise and needs prompt referral.** Childhood tumours of the brain and eye often present with a turned eye.

- **Never 'observe' a child with strabismus** – it is very rare for a child to 'grow out of it'. Delay in ophthalmic referral can result in permanent visual loss from amblyopia ('lazy eye').

SQUINT TERMINOLOGY

There are many terms related to squint. A few of the basic ones are:

- Terms for normal eye movements:
    - adduction: eye looking in towards the nose
    - abduction: eye looking out towards the ear
    - elevation: eye looking up
    - depression: eye looking down.
- Horizontal squints:
    - eye turned in: esotropia
    - eye turned out: exotropia
    - both of these can be constant or intermittent; they can always affect one eye or alternate between the two eyes.
- Vertical squints:
    - one eye higher: hypertropia
    - one eye lower: hypotropia.

OPHTHALMIC MANAGEMENT

The basic management of childhood squint by ophthalmologists is step-wise:

1. Exclude a serious underlying cause.
2. Correct refractive error, if present, with glasses.
3. If one eye is persistently turned and has poor vision from amblyopia, patch the 'straight' eye to force the turned eye to form normal connections with the brain's visual cortex and reverse amblyopia. Patching might be needed part-time for months or years, and requires close ophthalmic supervision.
4. Once maximum visual improvement in the amblyopic eye has been attained, perform squint surgery to align the eyes. Patching might need to continue after surgery.

DIAGNOSTIC FLOWCHART 6.1: TURNED EYE IN CHILDREN

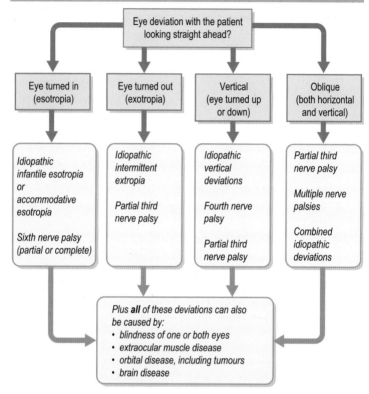

Examination 'clues' to the cause:
- **restriction** of eye movements in any direction (both eyes don't move fully in all directions): brain, nerve, muscle or orbit disease is possible. Restriction of movement can be very subtle and difficult to detect (e.g. in fourth nerve palsy or partial third or sixth nerve palsies)
- **enlarged pupil** that reacts poorly to light: suspect third nerve palsy
- **ptosis** (drooping upper lid): suspect third nerve palsy or muscle disease
- **proptosis** (eyeball pushed forwards): orbital inflammation or tumour
- **red eye**: orbital inflammation or tumour
- **head tilted** towards one shoulder: suspect fourth nerve palsy
- **other neurologic signs**: brain or nerve disease

APPROACH TO A CHILD WITH A 'TURNED EYE'

ASK

- How and when was the problem noticed?
- Which eye turns?
- Is the turn constant or intermittent?
- Do the parents think the child can see? (as appropriate for age) – most children can:
  - keep eye contact with their parent at age 6 weeks
  - show interest in bright objects at 2–3 months
  - fix and follow objects with their eyes at 3–4 months.

LOOK FOR

1. **Can the child see**, and can they see equally out of both eyes?
2. If there is an eye 'turn' (squint, strabismus), what **direction** is the deviation?
3. Does each eye **move fully** in all directions?
4. Is there anything wrong with the **eyes** apart from the squint (e.g. cataract, retinal tumour, optic nerve disease)?
5. Is there anything wrong with the **child** apart from the squint (e.g. developmental delay, neurological or metabolic disease)?

CAN THE CHILD SEE WITH BOTH EYES OPEN?

- Observe the child while you're talking to the parents.
- 3–4 months or older:
  - can the child fix and follow a toy?
  - will the child pick up small sweets or toys?
- Older children:
  - can the child identify small pictures or read the visual acuity chart?

DO THE TWO EYES SEE EQUALLY WELL?

- Try to repeat the above tests with one eye covered at a time (this is often difficult).
- Does the child object equally to covering each eye? (he or she won't mind having a blind eye covered as much as a 'good' eye).

EYE ALIGNMENT LOOKING STRAIGHT AHEAD

- Observation.
  - with the child looking at you or a torch, does one eye seem to be turned? In which direction?

LOOK FOR

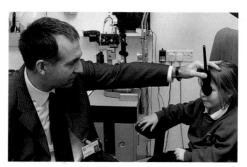

Fig. 6.1 The cover test.

- **Cover test** (this can be difficult in young children) (Fig. 6.1):
  - with the child looking straight ahead at an interesting target, cover the right eye (you can use your hand, a piece of cardboard, etc.) – look at the left eye the whole time
  - **if the left eye moves when you cover the right eye, the left eye is the turned eye**
  - if it moves out, it was turned in (esotropia)
  - if it moves in, it was turned out (exotropia)
  - if it moves down, it was turned up (hypertropia) and so on
  - uncover the right eye
  - now cover the left eye – look at the right eye the whole time
  - **if the right eye moves when you cover the left eye, the right eye is the turned eye.**

EYE MOVEMENTS (3–4 MONTHS OR OLDER)
- With both eyes open, have the child track a slow-moving toy from side to side and up and down.
- Try to repeat this one eye at a time, with the other eye covered with the parent's hand or a patch.
- Does each eye move fully in all directions?

RED REFLEX
- If the red reflex is absent on one or both sides, cataract, retinoblastoma tumour or other serious disease could be present and requires urgent referral.

RELATIVE AFFERENT PUPILLARY DEFECT (RAPD)

- See p. 25 for details of how to test for this. The presence of a relative afferent pupillary defect is indicative of serious retinal or optic nerve disease.

OPHTHALMOSCOPY

- Try to see the optic discs: are they normal? Is there swelling?
- This is often difficult in young children.
- In general, don't use dilating eye drops for children; special concentrations of drops will be used by the ophthalmologist if necessary.

IDIOPATHIC CHILDHOOD DEVIATIONS

- These are a collection of common childhood strabismus syndromes of unknown cause, which usually occur in otherwise healthy children.
- **A child presenting with any of these syndromes requires semi-urgent ophthalmic referral.**
- They are **diagnoses of exclusion,** after underlying eye, nerve and brain disease have been looked for and ruled out (this can usually be done clinically by an experienced ophthalmologist, but sometimes other tests are necessary).

IDIOPATHIC ESOTROPIA (ONE EYE IS TURNED IN)

- Idiopathic infantile esotropia ('congenital' esotropia) (Fig. 6.2):
  - first noticed by parents before 6 months of age
  - usually there is no significant refractive error
  - correction with surgery.
- Accommodative esotropia:
  - onset usually 2–4 years of age
  - hypermetropic ('long-sighted') refractive error
  - prescription of glasses may partly or completely correct the squint.
- Diseases that can *mimic* idiopathic esotropia:
  - partial or complete unilateral or bilateral sixth nerve palsy
  - blind eye
  - brain disease.

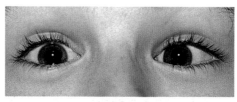

Fig. 6.2 Idiopathic infantile esotropia.

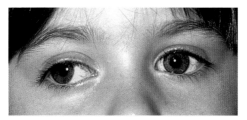

Fig. 6.3 Idiopathic childhood exotropia.

IDIOPATHIC INTERMITTENT EXOTROPIA (ONE EYE IS TURNED OUT) (Fig. 6.3)

- Onset as an intermittent deviation after 2 years of age.
- Correction with surgery if it becomes frequent or constant.
- Diseases that can mimic intermittent exotropia:
  - partial third nerve palsy (limited adduction of one eye)
  - blind eye
  - brain disease.

IDIOPATHIC VERTICAL DEVIATIONS

- These include dissociated vertical deviation and Brown's syndrome (please see one of the texts in 'Further reading' for details).
- Diseases that can mimic idiopathic vertical deviations:
  - partial third nerve palsy, fourth nerve palsy
  - blind eye
  - brain disease

OTHER CAUSES OF CHILDHOOD STRABISMUS

- Blind eyes in children tend to turn (often resulting in an esotropia or exotropia).
- Any of the causes of adult strabismus can also occur in children, for example:
  - brain tumours can present with any type of squint
  - orbital tumours can present with a squint
  - infectious or inflammatory disease result in third, fourth or sixth nerve palsies.
- Children can be born with a congenital palsy of the fourth nerve – this often presents as a head tilt (the child does this to compensate for the visual tilt produced by the palsy).

DOUBLE VISION IN ADULTS

OVERVIEW

Adults with a turned eye will present to you complaining of double vision (diplopia – seeing two images of everything). The only exceptions to this occur if there is poor vision in one eye, if the squint has been present since childhood or in complete third nerve palsy in which a complete ptosis occludes the eye.

Most adults with double vision have significant eye muscle, nerve or brain pathology. Examples include thyroid eye disease, myasthenia gravis, palsies of the ocular motor nerves and complex eye movement problems from brainstem disease. Third, fourth or sixth cranial nerve palsies are often 'ischaemic' (due to diabetes, hypertension or temporal arteritis) in the elderly, but cannot be assumed to be so without a careful work-up. In particular, partial or complete third nerve palsy in an adult is often due to an expanding cerebral arterial aneurysm, which could rupture and kill the patient unless diagnosed and operated on immediately. **Every adult with new-onset double vision requires urgent ophthalmic referral.**

Adults (and children over the age of 9) do *not* develop amblyopia ('lazy eye') if one eye is constantly turned. However, constant double vision can be very annoying, makes driving illegal and often interferes with the patient's life.

Double vision in adults *Critical points*

- **New-onset double vision** in a patient of any age is a life-threatening cerebral aneurysm until proven otherwise – **all require urgent (same-day) ophthalmic referral**.
- **Never prescribe spectacle prism** for double vision of unknown cause unless the patient has been assessed by an ophthalmologist. Brain tumours are a common cause of gradual-onset diplopia.
- **If a patient over 50 has transient or persisting double vision, ask about symptoms of temporal arteritis (see p. 216).**

DIAGNOSTIC FLOWCHART 6.2: DOUBLE VISION IN ADULTS

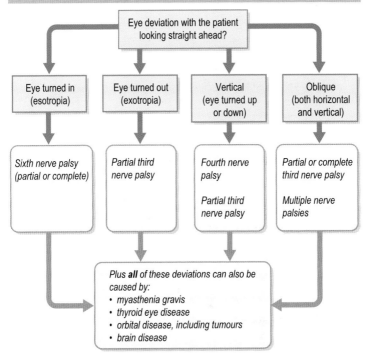

Examination 'clues' to the cause:
- **restriction** of eye movements in any direction (both eyes don't move fully in all directions): brain, nerve, muscle or orbit disease is possible. Restriction of movement can be very subtle and difficult to detect (e.g. in fourth nerve palsy or partial third or sixth nerve palsies)
- **enlarged pupil** that reacts poorly to light: suspect third nerve palsy
- **ptosis** (drooping upper lid): suspect third nerve palsy or myasthenia gravis
- **lid retraction** (upper lid too high): thyroid eye disease
- **proptosis** (eyeball pushed forwards): thyroid eye disease, orbital inflammation or tumour
- **red eye**: active thyroid eye disease, orbital inflammation
- **head tilted** towards one shoulder: suspect fourth nerve palsy
- **weakness of facial or body muscles**: myasthenia gravis
- **other neurologic signs**: brain or nerve disease

OPHTHALMIC MANAGEMENT

The basic management of adult squint by ophthalmologists is step-wise:

1. Exclude a serious underlying cause.
2. Treat the underlying cause if possible.
3. If no treatable cause is found (e.g. in 'ischaemic' sixth nerve palsy), relieve the double vision while awaiting recovery – by patching or prism spectacle lens. If no recovery in 6–12 months, eye muscle squint surgery may be considered.

APPROACH TO AN ADULT WITH DOUBLE VISION

ASK

PRESENTING COMPLAINT

- When was the double vision first noticed?
- Was the onset sudden or gradual? (sudden onset is often ischaemic; gradual onset might be a tumour, although there are exceptions to this).
- Is it constant or does it vary depending on time of day? (if worse at night or when tired: could be myasthenia).

SPECIFIC QUESTIONING

- Is there pain in or around the eye?
- Are there any neurological symptoms, e.g. headache, vertigo, limb weakness or numbness?
- Are there any symptoms of systemic myasthenia gravis? (e.g. drooping eyelids late in the day, limb muscle weakness, problems swallowing or breathing).
- If the patient is over 50, check for symptoms of temporal arteritis. (see p. 216).

PREVIOUS MEDICAL HISTORY

- Risk factors for 'ischaemic' nerve palsy, e.g. diabetes, hypertension, smoker? (however, this does *not* mean that a nerve palsy found in such a patient *is* ischaemic).

LOOK FOR

1. Does the patient have **normal vision** in each eye?
2. Which eye is turned, and what **direction** is the turn with the patient looking straight ahead?
3. Do both eyes **move fully** in all directions?
4. Is there anything wrong with the **eyes** apart from the squint?

5. Is there anything wrong with the **patient** apart from the squint? Ask whether the patient has any other neurological symptoms; if so, do a full neurological examination.

VISUAL ACUITY

VISUAL FIELDS

⬤ Pituitary tumours can present with a squint (and a bitemporal hemianopia on visual field testing).

ORBITAL SIGNS

⬤ Proptosis (eyeball pushed forwards) – in thyroid eye disease and orbital tumours.
⬤ Conjunctival redness and swelling – in acute thyroid eye disease or other inflammatory disease.

EYELIDS

⬤ Ptosis (drooping upper eyelid) can be a sign of:
  ▶ partial or complete third nerve palsy
  ▶ myasthenia gravis
  ▶ Horner's syndrome (mild ptosis only)
  ▶ orbit disease (e.g. tumour – usually also with proptosis)
⬤ Eyelid retraction (upper lid too high; +/– lower lid too low):
  ▶ common in thyroid eye disease (giving the eye(s) a 'staring' appearance).

PUPIL SIZE AND REACTION TO LIGHT AND DARK

⬤ A large pupil that constricts poorly to light can be a sign of third nerve palsy.
⬤ A small pupil that dilates poorly in the dark can be a sign of Horner's syndrome.

RELATIVE AFFERENT PUPILLARY DEFECT (RAPD)

⬤ If present, retinal or optic nerve disease is present.

EYE ALIGNMENT AND MOVEMENT

⬤ Assess as described for 'childhood squints' (see p. 133).

OPHTHALMOSCOPY

⬤ Are the optic discs normal? Is there bilateral optic disc swelling? (could be a brain tumour).

SYSTEMIC AND NEUROLOGIC EXAMINATION

⬤ As needed.

BRAIN DISEASES

Brain tumours, multiple sclerosis (MS) and stroke are all common causes of double vision in adults. Diseases affecting the brainstem can cause several types of strabismus: for example:

- **Internuclear ophthalmoplegia (INO):**
  - right internuclear ophthalmoplegia: when the patient tries to look left the right eye can't move all the way in to the nose (adduction deficit); the left eye moves out towards the left ear normally but oscillates horizontally (abducting nystagmus)
  - vice versa for left internuclear ophthalmoplegia.
- **Gaze palsies:**
  - these are limitations of voluntary eye movement to one side, e.g. neither eye may be able to look to the right.

NERVE DISEASES

The **third, fourth and sixth cranial nerves** between them supply all six extraocular muscles of each eye:

- Third nerve: superior rectus, inferior rectus, medial rectus and inferior oblique; plus the levator muscle (which elevates the upper lid) and the pupil constrictor muscle (which makes the pupil constrict to light).
- Fourth nerve: superior oblique.
- Sixth nerve: lateral rectus.

THIRD NERVE PALSY

CAUSES

- Compression of the third nerve by aneurysm or tumour.
  - can occur in adults of *any age*
  - an expanding **posterior communicating artery aneurysm** is a common cause of partial or complete third nerve palsy – **this can kill the patient within hours of onset of the double vision** if it is not detected and treated before it ruptures (Fig. 6.4).
- Ischaemia of the nerve: overall the most common cause of third nerve palsy in adults.
  - atherosclerosis, diabetes, hypertension
  - temporal arteritis (this is a less common but more serious cause – think of this in patients over age 50).

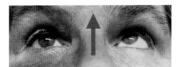
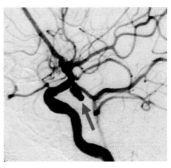

Fig. 6.4 Right partial third nerve palsy due to compression of the third nerve by a right posterior communicating artery aneurysm (right picture, arrow). The only abnormality on examination was decreased elevation of the right eye on looking up; other movements and the pupil were normal.

- Inflammation of the nerve: e.g. viral infections or post-viral autoimmune reaction.
- Raised intracranial pressure.
- Trauma.

SYMPTOMS

- Horizontal, vertical or oblique diplopia.
- In some patients, 'drooping' upper eyelid (ptosis) – if complete and occluding the eye, the patient will not complain of diplopia.

SIGNS

- A third nerve palsy can be partial (some function remains in one or more of the muscles supplied by the nerve) or complete (all function has been lost).
- A complete third nerve palsy is easy to diagnose.
- **Partial third nerve palsies can mimic other types of strabismus and be difficult to diagnose.**
- **Partial** third nerve palsy can show **one or more of:**
  - exotropia – with decreased adduction
  - vertical deviation (hypertropia or hypotropia) – decreased elevation or depression

- oblique deviation – a combination of exotropia and vertical deviation
- the upper lid may be normal or show ptosis (drooping upper lid)
- the pupil may be normal, slightly dilated, or very dilated (if dilated, it also reacts poorly to light).
- **Complete** third nerve palsy (Fig. 6.5) signs:
  - complete ptosis (eyelid completely closed)
  - eye deviated outwards (exotropia) and usually also slightly downwards (hypotropia)
  - the eye can't move 'up, down or in' at all
  - the pupil may be normal, or dilated and unreactive to light
- *Note:* 'pupil-sparing' third nerve palsies:
  - it used to be said that if an eye with a third nerve palsy had a normal pupil (rather than a dilated pupil, i.e. that if the nerve palsy was 'pupil sparing') the patient did not require neuroimaging because the cause was ischaemic and not compressive
  - however, aneurysms and tumours *can* cause 'pupil-sparing' third nerve palsies and partial progressive palsies, when the pupil is initially 'spared' but later involved
  - for this reason **all patients with third nerve palsy should be urgently assessed by an ophthalmologist, regardless of the state of the pupil.**

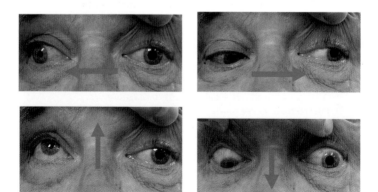

Fig. 6.5 Left complete left third nerve palsy: complete ptosis and inability to adduct, elevate or depress the left eye. In this case the left pupil was dilated and unreactive to light.

MANAGEMENT

- **Urgent ophthalmic referral** for careful examination +/− further investigation (including urgent neuroimaging to detect aneurysm or tumour if required).

FOURTH NERVE PALSY

SYMPTOMS

- Vertical, oblique or 'tilted' double vision.

SIGNS

- Fourth nerve palsy can be very difficult to detect clinically; most non-ophthalmologists say that it looks to them that the eyes 'move normally'. Often, the diagnosis cannot be made without careful examination (including cover test and prism measurements) by a practitioner experienced in eye-movement disorders.
- The patient will often have a head tilt to the side opposite the palsy.

CAUSES

- Idiopathic congenital.
- Trauma (often mild closed head injury without loss of consciousness).
- Compression – by a brain tumour.
- Ischaemia – atherosclerosis, hypertension, diabetes, or temporal arteritis.
- Inflammation or infection.

MANAGEMENT

- Urgent ophthalmic referral for further examination and investigation.

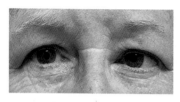
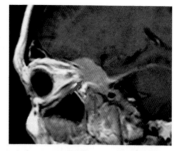
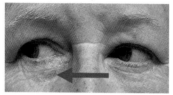
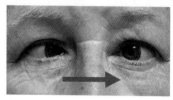

Fig. 6.6 Left sixth nerve palsy. Top left: a left esotropia looking straight ahead. Bottom pictures show that all eye movements are normal except that the left eye cannot abduct when patient tries to look left. This nerve palsy was the only clinical sign of a left sphenoidal meningioma (top right MRI scan, arrows).

SIXTH NERVE PALSY

SYMPTOMS

- Horizontal diplopia.

SIGNS

- Esotropia with limitation of abduction of the eye.

CAUSES

- Ischaemia (diabetes, hypertension, temporal arteritis).
- Compression by a brain tumour (Fig. 6.6).
- Inflammation.
- Trauma.
- Raised intracranial pressure of any cause can cause a unilateral or bilateral sixth nerve palsy.

MANAGEMENT

- All require urgent ophthalmic referral for further examination +/– investigation.

EYE MUSCLE DISEASES

- There are many diseases of the extraocular muscles, the commonest of which is thyroid eye disease.
- Myasthenia gravis is not strictly a disease of the muscles themselves (it is a disease of the neuromuscular junction), but is included here because it causes muscle dysfunction.
- **Both myasthenia and thyroid eye disease can mimic any pattern of strabismus.**
- Looking at the eyelids can help:
  - if the upper lid is retracted (too high), thyroid eye disease is likely
  - if the upper lid is drooping (ptosis – too low), myasthenia is a possibility.

MYASTHENIA GRAVIS

- Auto-antibodies attack the neuro-muscular junction.
- Drooping upper eyelid/s (ptosis) and/or double vision (diplopia) can occur.
- Often variable, changing from day to day and during each day (worse at night or when tired).
- The ptosis might increase if you ask the patient to look up at the ceiling for 2 minutes.
- Non-ophthalmic symptoms can include:
  - arm or leg weakness and easy fatigue
  - problems swallowing or breathing (symptoms of severe disease – can be fatal).
- Urgent ophthalmic referral.
- Managed in conjunction with a neurologist.

THYROID EYE DISEASE

- Thyroid eye disease (Fig. 6.7) is a common complication of Graves' disease (idiopathic hyperthyroidism).
- The eye disease seems to run a course independent to the thyroid disease, and occur before, during or after the period of hyperthyroidism.
- The clinical signs are due to enlargement and inflammation of the extraocular muscles and inflammation of the other orbital tissues.

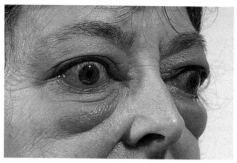

Fig. 6.7 Thyroid eye disease.

SYMPTOMS

- (Often) double vision.
- Visible change in eye appearance (the eyes seem more prominent due to lid retraction and proptosis).
- Discomfort/gritty eyes.
- (Rarely) blurred vision – this requires urgent assessment because it could be due to:
  - compressive optic neuropathy (the enlarged muscles compress the optic nerve at the orbital apex – severe proptosis does *not* have to be present for this to occur)
  - corneal exposure, if proptosis is severe.

SIGNS

One or more of:
- Any pattern of strabismus, with restriction of ocular movement in any direction (most commonly esotropia or hypotropia).
- Conjunctival swelling and redness.
- Eyelid swelling.
- Upper and lower eyelid retraction (gives a 'staring' appearance).
- Proptosis ('bulging' eye(s) – eyeballs pushed forwards).
- Signs of complications:
  - exposure corneal ulcer if severe proptosis
  - decreased visual acuity, decreased colour vision and relative afferent papillary defect if compressive optic neuropathy.

MANAGEMENT

- All patients with symptomatic thyroid eye disease need ophthalmic follow-up.
- **Any patient with Graves' disease complaining of *blurred*** (rather than just double) **vision requires urgent ophthalmic referral** to exclude compressive optic neuropathy.

ORBIT DISEASES

- Orbit tumours or inflammation of any cause can cause double vision.
- Proptosis (eyeball pushed forwards) is usually present but can be subtle or even absent.

CAUSES

- Infection, e.g. orbital cellulitis (see p. 189).
- Non-infectious orbital inflammation.
- Tumours:
  - benign or malignant, any age
  - can mimic inflammation or infection.

BLIND EYE

- Blind eyes can turn in adults, as well as in children.
- Although blind eyes in children can turn in or out, in adults they tend to turn out ('sensory exotropia'). The patient does not usually notice double vision because of the poor vision in the turned eye.

CHAPTER

ABNORMAL APPEARANCE
OF THE EYE OR EYELIDS

7

CHAPTER CONTENTS—*cont'd*

OVERVIEW

Patients sometimes present because they or their relatives have noticed an abnormal appearance of their eye. In other cases, you might incidentally notice an abnormality a patient is unaware of (e.g. unequal pupils) or your examination for a non-ophthalmic problem might reveal an abnormality in the eye (e.g. swollen optic discs on ophthalmoscopy in a patient with headaches).

Many of the conditions mentioned below are common and not serious. In a few, however, immediate recognition is essential. For instance, it is important that all practitioners can distinguish preseptal cellulitis from the rarer, sight- and life-threatening orbital cellulitis. This is not always easy on cursory examination, unless you know what to look for. Importantly, this clinical distinction requires no more sophisticated equipment than a visual acuity chart and a torch.

Abnormal eye or eyelid appearance **Critical points**

- **Every neonate should have their red reflexes checked** with a direct ophthalmoscope in a dark room, as part of their routine first physical examination.

- **A child with an absent red reflex or white pupil** has a retinoblastoma or cataract until proven otherwise – refer urgently.

- **A child or adult with severely swollen red eyelids on one side** has orbital cellulitis until proven otherwise – this is a sight- and life-threatening medical emergency.

- **If the patient can't blink, the cornea is in danger** – patients with facial nerve palsies or major facial burns need intensive lubricant eye ointment treatment, plus urgent ophthalmic consultation to prevent corneal ulceration.

- **Swollen optic discs can be the only sign of a brain tumour** – for this reason, every patient with headaches requires ophthalmoscopy as part of the routine examination, and urgent referral if disc swelling is found.

ABNORMAL EYE APPEARANCE

SPOT ON THE EYE SURFACE

DIAGNOSTIC FLOWCHART 7.1: SPOT ON THE EYE SURFACE

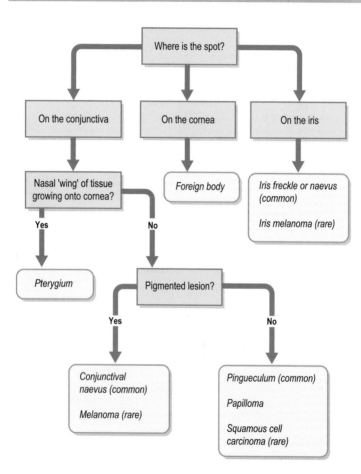

APPROACH TO A PATIENT WITH AN EYE SURFACE SPOT

Most incidentally noticed spots on the ocular surface are benign pingueculae, pterygia or naevi. Occasionally, however, malignancy can occur – the risk of malignancy increases if:

- The patient is middle-aged or elderly.
- The lesion is new.
- There is rapid growth in a pre-existing lesion.

ASK

- Duration?
- Growth?
- Other symptoms, e.g. pain, irritation, bleeding?

LOOK FOR (WITH MAGNIFICATION IF POSSIBLE):

- Location, colour of lesion.
- Thickness.
- Irregular margins.
- (Iris lesions): distorted pupil?

CONJUNCTIVAL SPOT

Benign conjunctival lesions

- Common in older teenagers and adults of all ages.
- Pingueculum (Fig 7.1, right):
  - small yellowish lump on the nasal or temporal sclera
  - does not require treatment.
- Conjunctival papilloma:
  - 'warty' soft mass anywhere on the conjunctiva
  - can be excised if causing irritation, but might recur.

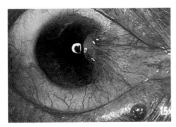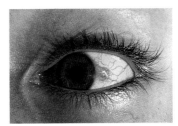

Fig. 7.1 Left, pterygium; right, pingueculum.

- Pterygium (Fig. 7.1, left):
  - wing-shaped fold of vascularised tissue growing from the nasal white sclera onto the clear cornea
  - excision is indicated only if it grows significantly and threatens the visual axis.
- Conjunctival naevus:
  - congenital lesions that might become rapidly pigmented at puberty
  - no treatment is needed except for cosmesis or on suspicion of malignant change (which is rare).

Malignant conjunctival lesions

- These are rare: malignant melanoma and squamous cell carcinoma (SCC).

CORNEAL SPOT

- Corneal foreign body.
- Pterygium extends from the conjunctiva onto the cornea (see above).

IRIS SPOT

- Iris naevi are small flat brown spots, visible in many normal eyes with close observation, and are harmless (Fig. 7.2).
- Iris melanomas are very rare. Suspicious signs include a raised iris mass or pupil distortion.

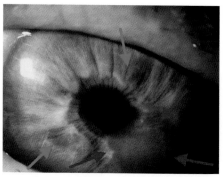

Fig. 7.2 Benign iris naevi (green arrows); malignant iris melanoma distorting the pupil (red arrows).

UNEQUAL PUPILS

DIAGNOSTIC FLOWCHART 7.2: UNEQUAL PUPILS

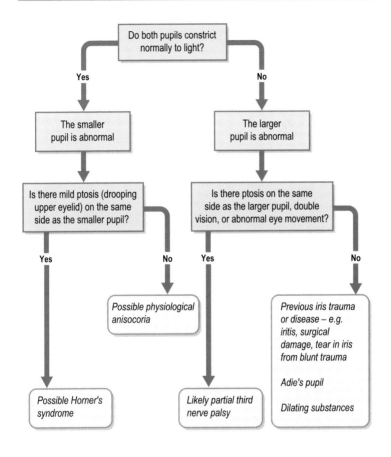

APPROACH TO A PATIENT WITH UNEQUAL PUPILS

Up to 20% of healthy people have slightly different-sized pupils on close observation. However, difference in pupil size (anisocoria) can also herald serious disease, such as Horner's syndrome or partial third nerve palsy due to brain disease. In these situations, the 'serious' abnormal pupil can often be identified by 'the company it keeps', for example:

- Horner's syndrome: abnormally small pupil plus mild (often subtle) ptosis (drooping upper lid)
- third nerve palsy: abnormally large pupil plus mild or severe ptosis and/or restriction of eye movement causing double vision.

Slightly abnormal sized pupils noted incidentally in a well patient, with no ptosis or double vision, normal eye examination and no headaches or neurological symptoms is unlikely to be serious.

Note: retinal or optic nerve disease can cause a relative afferent pupil defect on the 'swinging torch' test (see Chapter 1, p. 25) but does *not* cause different-sized pupils.

ASK

- How was the condition noticed?
- Duration (is it present in old photos)?
- History of eye trauma or eye disease?
- Is the patient using eye drops?
- Are there any visual symptoms:
  - double vision?
  - blurred vision?
- Any neurological symptoms? Headache?

LOOK FOR

- Look carefully at the pupils:
  - pupil size: in room light, with the patient staring at a distant target, estimate the size of each pupil – are they equal?
  - pupil reaction to light: darken the room, keep the patient staring into the distance, then briefly shine a bright torch onto one pupil – the normal reaction is a brisk constriction. Repeat for other pupil.
  - *Note*: this is just testing whether each pupil has a normal reaction to light. Don't confuse this with the 'swinging torch' test for

relative afferent pupil defect (RAPD), which is a separate test (see p. 25).

- Compare the upper lid height on both sides. Is there ptosis (drooping upper lid)?
  - mild ptosis: possible Horner's syndrome or partial third nerve palsy
  - moderate or severe ptosis: likely third nerve palsy.
- Test the eye movements:
  - limitation of eye movement? (possible partial third nerve palsy)
- Slit lamp examination: is there an abnormality of the iris itself?
  - irregular pupil margin, e.g. due to old trauma or iritis
  - different coloured iris in each eye (heterochromia). Congenital Horner's syndrome can cause the iris on the affected side to be lighter in colour than the fellow eye; chronic iritis can also cause this.

IRIS TRAUMA OR DISEASE

- Blunt trauma commonly causes 'traumatic mydriasis' – a dilated pupil that might have an irregular shape and/or constrict poorly to light.
- Slit lamp examination: might show tears in the pupil margin.
- Iris disease (e.g. current or previous iritis) can result in a poorly reactive large or small pupil, which might also be irregular in shape. Signs of previous iritis might also be visible on slit lamp examination.

PHYSIOLOGICAL ANISOCORIA

- Up to 20% of normal people have slightly unequal pupils.
- Both pupils constrict briskly to light and both dilate briskly when the light is turned off.

HORNER'S SYNDROME (Fig. 7.3)

SYMPTOMS

- Usually asymptomatic: the eyelid and pupil changes are usually noticed incidentally by a relative or examining practitioner.
- If the patient has neck pain or a recent history of head or neck trauma, suspect internal carotid artery dissection as the cause.

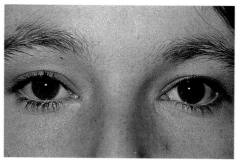

Fig. 7.3 Right Horner's syndrome: note mild right ptosis and right miosis (right pupil slightly smaller than left).

SIGNS

- Often subtle and difficult to detect.
- If unilateral:
  - mild ptosis ('drooping' upper lid)
  - miosis (abnormally small pupil that constricts briskly to light but dilates poorly in the dark).

MECHANISM

- Interruption of the sympathetic nerve supply to the eye and upper lid at any point in the head, neck or upper chest.
- Lack of sympathetic supply to the smooth muscle of the upper lid (Muller's muscle) causes the mild ptosis; lack of supply to the iris dilator muscle causes the small pupil.

CAUSES

- In infancy (the affected iris is usually lighter in colour):
  - idiopathic congenital
  - birth trauma.
- In children or adults:
  - head or neck tumour
  - trauma.
- In adults:
  - brainstem stroke
  - apical lung tumour (Pancoast syndrome)
  - dissecting aneurysm of the internal carotid artery.

MANAGEMENT

- **Refer urgently if onset was acute, there has been recent trauma or neck pain, or if neurological symptoms are present**; otherwise semi-urgent referral.
- All cases require careful ophthalmic and systemic examination to assess for serious causes, with imaging (if necessary) to look for a head or neck tumour or dissecting carotid aneurysm.
- All smokers with Horner's syndrome need a chest X-ray to check for apical lung cancer.
- However, in many patients no cause is found.

THIRD NERVE PALSY

See p. 142. It is exceptionally rare for one dilated pupil to be the only sign of partial third nerve palsy; there is usually also diplopia due to motility restriction (although this might become apparent only if the patient looks up, down or in) and/or ptosis.

ADIE'S PUPIL (Fig. 7.4)

- Possibly a viral infection of the orbital ciliary ganglion causing lack of parasympathetic supply to the eye. The iris sphincter muscle (which causes pupil constriction) is paralysed, resulting in a dilated pupil.
- Unilateral (less commonly bilateral).
- Occurs in otherwise well patients.

SYMPTOMS

- Mild blurring of vision, especially near (from paralysis of the ciliary muscle, which focuses the lens).
- Glare (from the dilated pupil).
- No double vision.

SIGNS

- Dilated pupil with very poor constriction to light but which constricts slowly when the patient is asked to look at a near target ('light-near dissociation').
- No ptosis, normal eye movements.

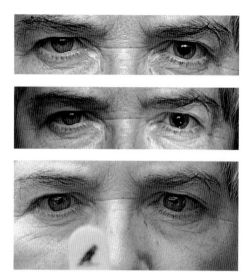

Fig. 7.4 Left Adie's tonic pupil. The left pupil is enlarged (top) and does not constrict to light (middle). However, it does constrict slowly when the patient focuses on a near target (bottom).

MANAGEMENT

- Ophthalmic referral to confirm diagnosis.
- Reading glasses might be necessary; sunglasses should be worn outside.

DILATING SUBSTANCES

- Inadvertent or intentional use of dilating eye drops.

OTHER CAUSES OF ABNORMAL PUPILS

- Argyll-Robertson pupils:
  - both pupils are small, irregular and poorly reactive to light (but may still constrict to near).
  - causes: neurosyphilis, diabetes, alcoholism.

WHITE PUPIL AND/OR NO RED REFLEX

DIAGNOSTIC FLOWCHART 7.3: WHITE PUPIL AND/OR NO RED REFLEX

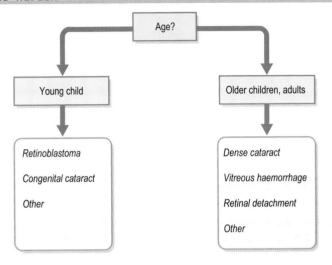

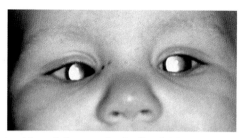

Fig. 7.5 Bilateral loss of the normal red reflex (with an abnormal 'white' reflex) in a child with bilateral retinoblastoma.

Most patients in whom this is incidentally noted are children (Fig. 7.5).

- Parents may notice that one or both pupils are white or grey, rather than black.
- An examining practitioner may notice that one or both eyes do not show the normal 'red reflex' reflection on testing with an ophthalmoscope in a dark room.
- Occasionally the parents may report the lack of a red reflex in one eye on looking at family flash photographs of the child.

The detection of a white pupil or abnormal red reflex in a child is important because:

- it can be a sign of serious disease – e.g. intraocular malignant retinoblastoma
- the cause of the abnormality (e.g. congenital cataract) can block the passage of light through the eye, and cause the affected eye(s) to become blind from amblyopia if not treated urgently.

Looking carefully for a red reflex is one of the most critical steps in examining any child's eyes (see p. 30 for the technique).

NYSTAGMUS (CONTINUALLY MOVING EYES)

DIAGNOSTIC FLOWCHART 7.4: NYSTAGMUS (CONTINUALLY MOVING EYES)

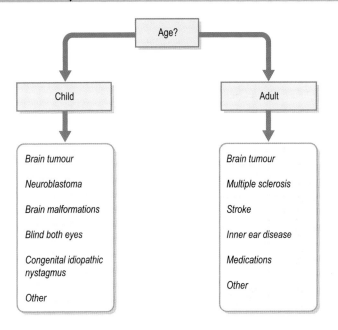

Nystagmus is a continuous rhythmic side-to-side, up-and-down or rotary oscillation of the eyes.

PRESENTATION

- Children who have nystagmus might be brought for assessment because their parents have noticed the abnormal eye movement.
- Adults with new-onset nystagmus often present complaining of vertigo or other neurological symptoms, with the eye movements being noticed incidentally on examination.

CAUSES

- Congenital nystagmus (noted at birth or in the first few months of life):
  - bilateral blindness (congenital retinal or optic nerve disease; anterior visual pathway tumour)
  - congenital idiopathic nystagmus (the eyes and the child are otherwise normal; the only abnormality is the nystagmus).
- Acquired nystagmus (any age):
  - inner ear disease
  - vestibulocochlear (eighth) nerve tumour
  - brainstem or cerebellar stroke, multiple sclerosis, tumour.

MANAGEMENT

- Any child or adult who presents with unexplained nystagmus must be presumed to have serious eye or brain disease until proven otherwise and referred for urgent assessment.

PROPTOSIS (EYE(S) PUSHED FORWARDS)

DIAGNOSTIC FLOWCHART 7.5: PROPTOSIS (EYE(S) PUSHED FORWARDS)

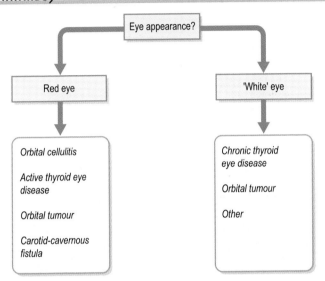

Eye appearance?

Red eye

Orbital cellulitis

Active thyroid eye disease

Orbital tumour

Carotid-cavernous fistula

'White' eye

Chronic thyroid eye disease

Orbital tumour

Other

PRESENTATION

- Patients might notice that one or both eyes appear more prominent ('staring' or 'bulging') than usual.
- Sometimes double vision and/or blurred vision.

CAUSES

In children:
- Proptosis is rare in children, and always serious.
- Orbital cellulitis (see p. 189).
- Orbital tumour.

In adults:
- Thyroid eye disease (see p. 147) is the most common cause of both unilateral and bilateral proptosis.
- Orbital cellulitis.
- Orbital tumour.

- Autoimmune orbital inflammation.
- Carotid–cavernous fistula (high-pressure arterial blood from the internal carotid artery flows into the orbit, causing proptosis which 'pulses' with each heartbeat).

MANAGEMENT

- All patients presenting with proptosis require urgent referral to exclude serious orbital disease.

ABNORMAL OPTIC DISC ON OPHTHALMOSCOPY

DIAGNOSTIC FLOWCHART 7.6: ABNORMAL OPTIC DISC ON OPHTHALMOSCOPY

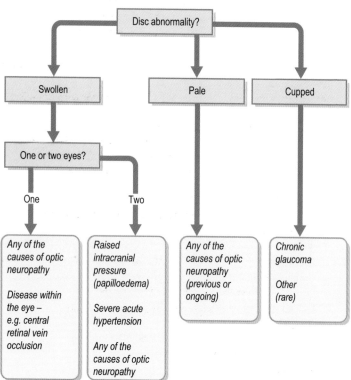

APPROACH TO A PATIENT WITH ABNORMAL OPTIC DISC(S)

The 'optic disc' (also called the 'optic nerve head') is the site where the optic nerve connects to the back of the eyeball. This may be noted to be abnormal during examination of a patient complaining of blurred vision, or sometimes incidentally during a routine eye check.

Ophthalmoscopy should be part of the routine examination of every patient complaining of headache or other neurologic symptoms, as early in the course of brain tumours bilateral swollen optic discs may be the only abnormal physical finding.

ASK

- Is there any blurred vision or transient loss of vision?
- Is there headache or other neurological symptoms?
- Does the patient have a family history of glaucoma?

LOOK FOR

- Visual acuity.
- Colour vision: in many optic neuropathies, colour perception is affected earlier and more severely than visual acuity.
  - Ishihara colour plates (if available; see p. 35)
  - ask the patient to compare the 'redness' of a red object viewed by each eye in turn: if one eye has optic nerve disease, the object's colour will often appear 'less deeply red' or 'washed out'.
- Visual fields to confrontation.
- 'Swinging torch' test for relative afferent pupil defect (RAPD) (see p. 25).
- Bilateral swollen discs:
  - is the blood pressure normal? (malignant hypertension can cause disc swelling)
  - is the systemic neurological examination normal?

In general, optic disc appearance may be classified as:
1. normal
2. swollen
3. pale ('optic atrophy')
4. 'cupped'
5. or have some other abnormality.

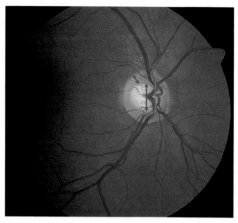

Fig. 7.6 Normal optic disc. Green arrow, total disc height; red arrow, central 'cup'; blue arrow, 'rim'; cup–disc ratio = green arrow height divided by red arrow height = approximately 0.5 in this case.

THE NORMAL OPTIC DISC

The normal optic disc (Fig. 7.6) is flat, pink and has a central pale excavated 'cup' that is usually less than half as wide as the disc itself. The ratio between the cup and the disc (the cup–disc ratio: see p. 32) is usually equal to or less than 0.5.

SWOLLEN OPTIC DISC(S)

SIGNS

- Normal or abnormal visual acuity and visual field.
- There might or might not be a relative afferent pupil defect.
- The swollen disc(s) (Fig. 7.7) have:
  - if mild swelling: blurred outer margins (not the normal clear margins)
  - if moderate or severe swelling: an elevated dome shape (rather than being flat as is normal) and dilated retinal veins; the normally clear disc vessels become partly obscured by swollen nerve fibres
  - there might be fine haemorrhages on and adjacent to severely swollen discs.

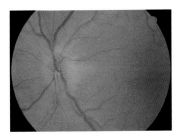
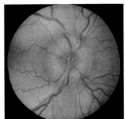
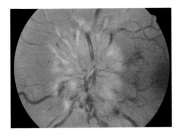

Fig. 7.7 Top left, mild disc swelling; top right, moderate disc swelling; bottom, severe disc swelling.

CAUSES

TWO SWOLLEN DISCS

- **Raised intracranial pressure** due to brain tumour, traumatic brain oedema, intracranial haemorrhage or other causes. Bilateral swollen discs as a result of *proven* raised intracranial pressure is called *papilloedema* (*note*: papilloedema is not a generic term for all cases of disc swelling).
- Severe acute hypertension.
- Almost any of the causes of acute or chronic optic neuropathy (see pp. 54 and 70).

ONE SWOLLEN DISC

- Disease within the eye, e.g. central retinal vein occlusion.
- Almost any of the causes of acute or chronic optic neuropathy.

MANAGEMENT

- **Refer urgently (to be seen the same day)** because urgent neuro-imaging might be required.

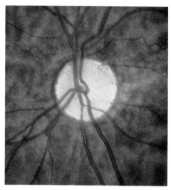

Fig. 7.8 Pale disc (optic atrophy).

- If disc swelling is bilateral: measure the blood pressure. However, even if severe hypertension is found it cannot be assumed to be the cause; the patient still needs imaging.

PALE OPTIC DISC(S) (OPTIC ATROPHY)

SIGNS

- Decreased visual acuity, colour vision loss or visual field loss in the affected eye(s) (although this might be subtle).
- The disc(s) are flat and paler than normal (Fig. 7.8).

CAUSES

- **Any** of the many causes of acute or slowly progressive optic neuropathy can result in pale optic disc(s).
- The disease damaging the optic nerve(s) might have been a sudden event many years previously or there might be ongoing active damage (e.g. from a compressive tumour).
- The disc might previously have been swollen or might have looked normal but slowly turned pale.

MANAGEMENT

- **Refer semi-urgently for investigation** unless an ophthalmologist has previously determined a definite cause (the patient could have an undiagnosed orbit or pituitary tumour).

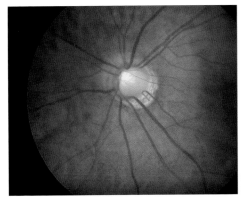

Fig. 7.9 Glaucomatous optic disc showing 'cupping'.

'CUPPED' OPTIC DISC(S)

- Usually caused by chronic glaucoma (Fig. 7.9).
- Symptoms are usually absent until the disease is very advanced (hence the need for routine population screening).

SIGNS

- Enlargement and deepening of the central cup, thinning of the pink disc rim, increased cup–disc ratio (see p. 32).
- If due to mild to moderate chronic glaucoma:
  - visual acuity is usually normal
  - intraocular pressure might be elevated (or normal in cases of 'normal tension glaucoma').

MANAGEMENT

- Ophthalmic referral for further investigation and/or treatment of glaucoma.
- The early identification of glaucoma by regular screening is important, as treatment can prevent later irreversible loss of central vision.

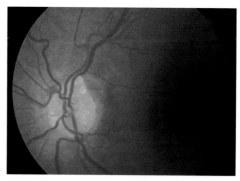

Fig. 7.10 Optic disc drusen.

OTHER OPTIC DISC ABNORMALITIES

These (usually harmless) abnormalities can be mistaken for optic disc swelling.

Degenerative changes

OPTIC DISC 'DRUSEN' (Fig. 7.10)

- Degenerative changes within the nerve head that sometimes mimic optic disc swelling.
- Drusen can be visible (producing a lumpy appearance), or hidden deep in the optic disc tissue.
- The patient usually remains asymptomatic and has good vision.

Congenital anomalies

MYELINATED NERVE FIBRES (Fig. 7.11)

- A harmless congenital anomaly in which retinal nerve fibres (usually at the edge of the optic disc) are white and opaque, rather than transparent.
- This gives the disc a white, feathery border on one or more sides.

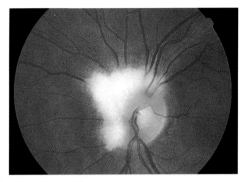

Fig. 7.11 Myelinated nerve fibres.

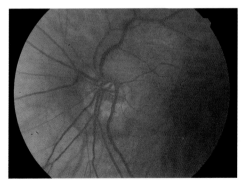

Fig. 7.12 Tilted optic discs.

'TILTED' DISCS (Fig. 7.12)

- Oblique, tilted discs are commonly seen in patients with severe myopia or astigmatism.

'CROWDED' DISCS

- These discs are small and raised, and may be mistaken for swollen discs.
- Often seen in longsighted (hypermetropic) patients.

ABNORMAL RETINAL OR OPTIC DISC BLOOD VESSELS ON OPHTHALMOSCOPY

Abnormal retinal blood vessels can be seen during eye examination for blurred vision or other symptoms, or detected during routine or screening eye examinations. Abnormal new vessels grow (and might bleed) in proliferative diabetic retinopathy; the existing retinal vessels can take on an abnormal appearance in chronic hypertension.

PROLIFERATIVE DIABETIC RETINOPATHY (Fig. 7.13)

This is the growth of abnormal retinal blood vessels due to diabetes.

SYMPTOMS

- Usually none (normal vision) until the vessels bleed – this is why regular screening examinations are needed.
- Bleeding can cause the sudden appearance of new floating spots in the patient's vision.

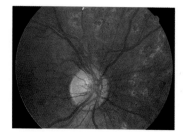 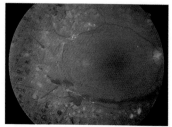

Fig. 7.13 Left, new vessels on the disc; right, peripheral new vessels (blue arrows), some of which have bled. Also visible are old laser treatment scars (scattered yellow and black spots).

SIGNS

- Abnormal new vessels on the optic disc and/or the retina. Initially, these might be very fine and difficult to see.
- If advanced, the new vessels appear as fan-shaped fronds, and often extend into the vitreous.
- **A direct ophthalmoscope is good at detecting disc new vessels but is *not* adequate to exclude new vessels elsewhere in the retina because of its small field of view.**
- If advanced, vitreous haemorrhage or retinal detachment might be present.
- Other signs of diabetic retinopathy are always present:
  - retinal haemorrhages and microaneurysms
  - hard exudates and cotton-wool spots.

MANAGEMENT

- **Regular routine eye screening of *all* diabetic patients.**
- Urgent ophthalmic referral for laser treatment if new diabetic vessels are suspected.

HYPERTENSIVE RETINOPATHY

Changes in the retina due to hypertension depend on the severity and duration of the raised blood pressure, and on the age of the patient.

Chronic mild to moderate hypertension

SYMPTOMS

- Usually none.

SIGNS ON OPHTHALMOSCOPY (BOTH EYES)

- Irregularity and narrowing of the retinal arteries
- 'A-V nipping': the arteries cause focal narrowing (nipping) of the retinal veins where they cross them (Fig. 7.14).

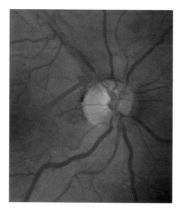

Fig. 7.14 'A-V nipping' (arrow).

MANAGEMENT

- Control blood pressure.
- **Patients with hypertension do *not* require regular eye screening** (unless they also have diabetes) because hypertensive retinopathy itself rarely causes vision problems.
- Poorly controlled chronic hypertension is a risk factor for many eye diseases, including retinal vascular occlusions, ischaemic optic neuropathy and worsening of diabetic retinopathy.

Severe acute hypertension

SYMPTOMS

- Vision might be normal or blurred.
- Headache or other neurological symptoms are common.

SIGNS ON OPHTHALMOSCOPY (BOTH EYES)

- Retinal haemorrhages and yellow hard exudates might occur.
- Bilateral optic disc swelling can occur.

MANAGEMENT

- Urgent admission to a medical unit for investigation and treatment.

ABNORMAL EYELID APPEARANCE

EYELID LUMP

DIAGNOSTIC FLOWCHART 7.7: EYELID LUMP

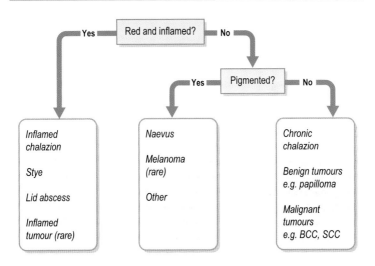

Most eyelid lumps in children are chalazia. These are non-infected inflammatory masses that almost always go away with time.

Chalazia can also occur in adults, but so can a range of benign and malignant lid tumours. The chance of malignancy increases if:

- The patient is elderly.
- There is progressive growth over months (compared with the sudden enlargement and fluctuating size of inflammatory lesions).
- There are clinical features of specific malignant lesions, e.g. basal cell carcinoma (BCC) or squamous cell carcinoma (SCC).

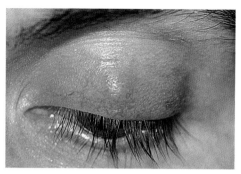

Fig. 7.15 Chalazion.

INFLAMMATORY EYELID LUMPS

Chalazion (Fig. 7.15)

- Non-infectious, granulomatous reaction to obstructed lid meibomian (lipid) glands.
- Can be mildly red and tender when acute and inflamed.
- When chronic, painless firm lumps deep in the upper or lower lids.

MANAGEMENT

- Do not require topical or oral antibiotics, as not infectious.
- Almost always resolve spontaneously.
- If not (in adults) incision and curette under local anaesthetic is usually curative.
- Treat conservatively in children as general anaesthetic is required for surgical treatment.

Stye (Fig. 7.16)

- A small pimple-like abscess surrounding an eyelash base.

TREATMENT

- Remove the central lash (this might allow discharge and resolution).
- If associated mild, localised (preseptal) cellulitis: oral antibiotics.

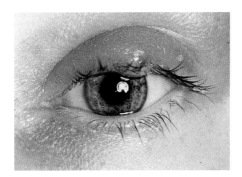

Fig. 7.16 Stye.

Lid abscess

- Fluctuant tender mass in the eyelid – can arise from a stye or other skin infection.

TREATMENT

- **Urgent ophthalmic referral (risk of progressing to orbital cellulitis).**

EYELID TUMOURS

- Any type of skin tumour can occur on the eyelid skin.

Benign

- Lid skin papilloma (Fig. 7.17, left):
  - small, wart-like growths
  - routine referral for excision if cosmetic problem.
- Sebaceous cysts (Fig 7.17, right):
  - small cysts filled with whitish material.
- Eyelid naevus:
  - small light- or dark-brown pigmented lump.

Malignant

APPEARANCE

BASAL CELL CARCINOMA
- Classic/nodular: rounded, pearly with telangiectatic edges (Fig. 7.18).
- Sclerosing/morpheaform: diffuse subcutaneous infiltration.

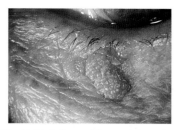 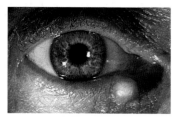

Fig. 7.17 Left, papilloma; right, sebaceous cyst.

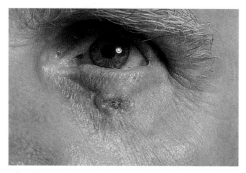

Fig. 7.18 Basal cell carcinoma (BCC) of the lower eyelid.

SQUAMOUS CELL CARCINOMA
- Rolled edges with central ulceration +/– a scaly keratin cover.

MALIGNANT MELANOMA
- Black flat or nodular lesion.
- New lesion or developing from pre-existing naevus.

MANAGEMENT
- **Refer urgently: the patient's life can be threatened if orbital extension of SCC occurs or a melanoma metastasises.**

ABNORMAL EYELID POSITION
DIAGNOSTIC FLOWCHART 7.8: ABNORMAL EYELID POSITION

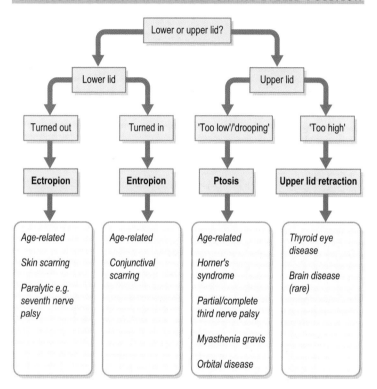

In general, lower eyelids can turn out (ectropion) or in (entropion). Upper lids can hang too low (ptosis) or too high (lid retraction).

Most cases of ectropion and entropion are age-related and, although a nuisance to the patient, aren't serious. Ptosis of the upper lid, however, needs more careful assessment, as dangerous conditions such as myasthenia and aneurysm (causing partial third nerve palsy) can present with a 'droopy' upper lid. Despite this, the majority of cases of adult ptosis are the result of harmless, age-related change. Upper lid retraction occurs most commonly with thyroid eye disease.

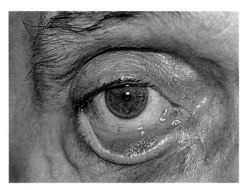

Fig. 7.19 Ectropion.

ECTROPION (Fig. 7.19)

- The lower lid is turned out.
- Often asymptomatic, but can cause watery eye (epiphora) or eye irritation.

CAUSES

- Age-related (most common).
- Scarring of the cheek region skin (from trauma, surgery or sun damage).
- Paralytic, e.g. seventh nerve palsy.

MANAGEMENT

- Routine referral for lid surgery if significant epiphora, irritation or cosmetic embarrassment.

ENTROPION (Fig. 7.20)

- The lower lid is turned in.
- Can result in the eyelashes abrading the cornea, causing foreign body sensation.

CAUSES

- Age-related (most common).
- Scarring of the lower lid conjunctiva.

MANAGEMENT

- Eyelashes abrading cornea: urgent referral.
- Otherwise routine referral for lid surgery.

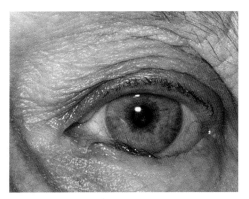

Fig. 7.20 Entropion.

PTOSIS (Fig. 7.21)

- The upper lid is drooping or is lower than normal.

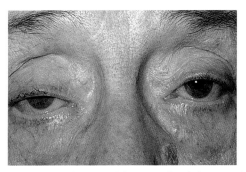

Fig. 7.21 Bilateral upper lid ptosis, right worse than left.

CAUSES

- Age-related (aponeurotic) due to stretching and thinning of the levator muscle or its connective tissue extension in the lid (the aponeurosis).
- Horner's syndrome.
- Partial third nerve palsy (mild or moderate ptosis).
- Complete third nerve palsy (complete ptosis).
- Myasthenia gravis.
- Orbital tumours or inflammation.
- Congenital idiopathic.

APPROACH TO A PATIENT WITH PTOSIS

- Unilateral or bilateral?
  - unilateral: any cause
  - bilateral: age-related or myasthenia most likely (it is rare for third nerve palsy or Horner's syndrome to be bilateral).
- Severity:
  - mild: any cause possible
  - moderate or severe: any cause except Horner's syndrome (it only produces a mild ptosis).
- Double vision and limited eye movements?
  - myasthenia or partial third nerve palsy.
- Abnormal pupil size on the side of the ptosis?
  - abnormally small pupil: possible Horner's syndrome
  - abnormally large pupil: possible partial third nerve palsy.
- Fatigability of the ptosis is highly suggestive of myasthenia:
  - the patient might report that the ptosis is worse at night or that it varies from day to day
  - myasthenia is likely if the degree of ptosis worsens markedly after prolonged upgaze for 2 minutes
  - a patient with myasthenia might also have problems swallowing or breathing, or arm or leg weakness.

MANAGEMENT

- Refer all cases of ptosis to an ophthalmologist to exclude serious underlying disease.
- Surgery if:
  - the drooping lid is obstructing vision (this can cause amblyopia in young children)
  - there is a significant cosmetic defect.

LID RETRACTION

- Almost always caused by thyroid eye disease (see p. 147); rarely due to midbrain disease.
- Nil required if not bothering the patient.
- Corrective eyelid surgery is possible after active thyroid eye disease has resolved, to improve cosmesis.

RED SWOLLEN EYELIDS ON ONE SIDE

DIAGNOSTIC FLOWCHART 7.9: RED SWOLLEN EYELIDS ON ONE SIDE

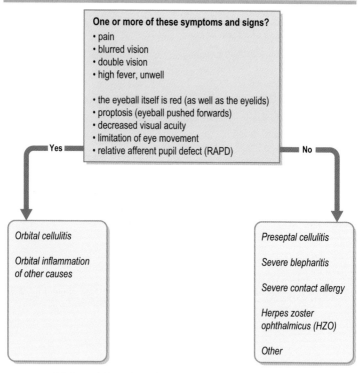

One or more of these symptoms and signs?
- pain
- blurred vision
- double vision
- high fever, unwell

- the eyeball itself is red (as well as the eyelids)
- proptosis (eyeball pushed forwards)
- decreased visual acuity
- limitation of eye movement
- relative afferent pupil defect (RAPD)

Yes

Orbital cellulitis

Orbital inflammation of other causes

No

Preseptal cellulitis

Severe blepharitis

Severe contact allergy

Herpes zoster ophthalmicus (HZO)

Other

A child or adult with unilateral, red, swollen eyelids could have a mild subcutaneous eyelid infection (preseptal cellulitis) or a severe life-threatening eye socket infection (orbital cellulitis). There are also other causes, such as herpes zoster ophthalmicus or severe allergy (see 'Skin rash around the eye', p. 191).

- Orbital cellulitis often requires many days' intravenous antibiotic treatment, plus drainage of an orbital abscess if identified on CT scan.
- Patients with preseptal cellulitis can often be safely treated by their general practitioner with oral antibiotics (except young children who are systemically unwell with the infection and who require admission).

ORBITAL CELLULITIS

A severe, sight- and life-threatening infection of the orbit (eye socket) soft tissues (Fig. 7.22). The infection is usually bacterial (rarely fungal). Complications include:
- Blindness from optic neuropathy.
- Death from meningitis or encephalitis.

SYMPTOMS

One or more of:
- Pain (often severe).
- Blurred vision.
- Double vision.
- Fever, malaise.

SIGNS

The presence of one or more of the following signs differentiates orbital cellulitis from preseptal cellulitis, which is less severe:
- The eyeball itself is red (as well as the eyelids).
- Proptosis (eyeball pushed forwards).
- Decreased visual acuity.
- Limitation of eye movement in one or more directions.
- Relative afferent pupil defect.
- High fever, unwell.

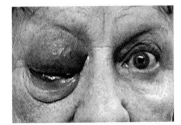 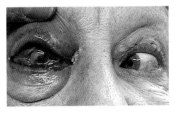

Fig. 7.22 Orbital cellulitis: left: severe eyelid swelling and redness; right: right eye redness, proptosis and lack of movement (the patient is trying to look to her right).

MANAGEMENT

- **Urgent ophthalmic referral for admission to hospital.**
- Urgent orbital CT scan (to exclude orbital or sinus abscesses, which are usually urgently drained with surgery).
- High-dose broad-spectrum intravenous antibiotics.

PRESEPTAL CELLULITIS

This is a much less dangerous infection of the subcutaneous tissue of the eyelids than orbital cellulitis. There is no extension into the orbit (Fig. 7.23).

SYMPTOMS AND SIGNS

- Mild to moderate eyelid swelling.
- None of the critical symptoms or signs of orbital cellulitis. Thus:
  - vision is normal
  - there is no diplopia
  - the patient has a full range of extraocular movements
  - there is no proptosis
  - there is no afferent pupil defect
  - the eyeball itself is not red
  - the patient is otherwise well – no fever.

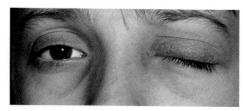

Fig. 7.23 Preseptal cellulitis: when the eyelid was lifted the left eye was white, had normal vision and moved fully in all directions.

MANAGEMENT

- **Small children who are unwell with a fever require urgent paediatric referral** to consider admission for intravenous antibiotic treatment (to decrease the risk of bacteraemia and systemic infection).
- Older children and adults who are otherwise well and have no signs of orbital cellulitis:
  - broad-spectrum oral antibiotic treatment
  - frequent review until resolved (refer urgently if worsen).

OTHER CAUSES OF RED SWOLLEN EYELIDS ON ONE SIDE

- Orbital inflammation of other causes.
- Herpes zoster ophthalmicus (see below).

SKIN RASH AROUND THE EYE

DIAGNOSTIC FLOWCHART 7.10: SKIN RASH AROUND THE EYE

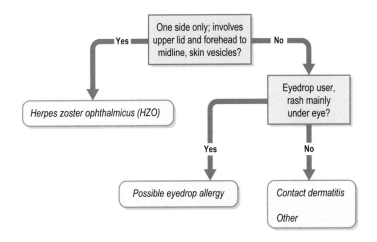

Most rashes around the eye are not serious and are often allergies. Herpes zoster ophthalmicus (HZO) is 'shingles' around the eye, the forehead above the eye and the side of the nose, and can be very painful. It can cause severe eyelid swelling and can thus mimic preseptal and (rarely) orbital cellulitis. **Patients with herpes zoster ophthalmicus require urgent ophthalmic referral** because the eyeball itself could become involved, with corneal ulcer or inflammation, iritis and other complications. Ocular complications of herpes zoster ophthalmicus can occur months or even years after the acute skin rash.

HERPES ZOSTER OPHTHALMICUS

This is caused by reactivation of the varicella-zoster (chickenpox/shingles) virus in the ophthalmic nerve (first division of the trigeminal nerve) distribution. It involves the eye, upper eyelid and forehead (Fig. 7.24).

SYMPTOMS

- Painful rash around the eye and forehead.
- The pain can start 1–2 days before the rash appears.
- Symptoms of eye complications might be present.

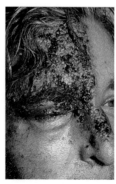

Fig. 7.24 Herpes zoster ophthalmicus.

SIGNS

RASH
- Vesicular.
- Red.
- Stops at the vertical midline of the nose and forehead.

SIGNS OF OCULAR COMPLICATIONS
- Decreased visual acuity.
- Corneal ulcers and haze, iritis, glaucoma, optic neuritis, restricted eye movements.

MANAGEMENT

- **Start oral antiviral treatment as soon as the diagnosis is made** as this reduces the length and severity of the episode and decreases the risk of ophthalmic complications.
- **Urgent referral to monitor for ophthalmic complications.**
- Eye complications (e.g. iritis and glaucoma) can occur many months after the rash has resolved.

CONTACT ALLERGIC RASH

- If the patient has an allergy to eyedrops, rash often on the lower eyelid skin (where the eyedrops would run).
- Thickened, erythematous, scaly skin.

MANAGEMENT

- Withdraw or change eye drop (consult the prescribing ophthalmologist).
- Mild topical steroid cream to skin (short term only).

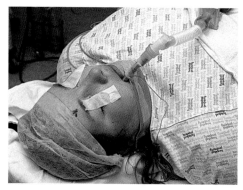

Fig. 7.25 Taping the eyelids shut to protect the corneas during general anaesthetic.

PATIENT CAN'T CLOSE THE EYELIDS

The main reasons why the eyelids may not close are:
- Seventh (facial) nerve palsy of any cause.
- Weak orbicularis muscle, e.g. myasthenia.
- Unconscious patient.
- Loss of eyelid tissue, e.g. severe facial burns.

A cornea not regularly lubricated with eyelid blinking will ulcerate and sight could be lost as a result. **Corneal ulceration** due to exposure is a rapid process, and **can occur within 24 hours** of the onset of the lid problem. Hence **any patient with an exposed cornea due to poor lid closure requires *urgent* ophthalmic referral**. The risk of ulceration is even greater if the cornea is numb (from fifth nerve palsy) as well as exposed.

   If an unconscious patient is under your care, you must ensure that the eyelids are closed at all times (e.g. tape the lids (Fig. 7.25) at the start of any general anaesthetic) or use frequent eye lubricants if you cannot close the eyelids (e.g. severe burns in intensive care).

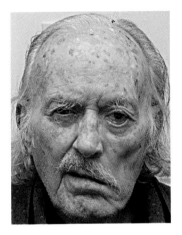
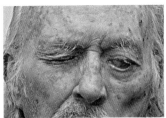

Fig. 7.26 Left seventh nerve palsy. Left, the patient is attempting to smile; right, the patient is attempting to close both eyes.

SEVENTH NERVE PALSY ('FACIAL PALSY') (Fig. 7.26)

CAUSES

- **Caution: not all seventh nerve palsies are 'Bell's palsy'!**
- Infections (e.g. herpes zoster).
- Inflammation (e.g. sarcoidosis).
- Ischaemia (e.g. diabetes).
- Tumours (e.g. acoustic neuroma, parotid tumours).
- Trauma.
- Idiopathic:
    - after the above diseases have been excluded by careful examination and/or investigations, acute idiopathic seventh nerve palsy with no other neurological symptoms or signs is called 'Bell's palsy'.

Seventh nerve palsy does not cause drooping of the upper lid (ptosis). The brow and face will droop but the upper lid does not (the upper lid levator muscle is supplied by the third nerve, not the seventh nerve).

MANAGEMENT

- **Urgent referral for ophthalmic assessment.**
- Acute ophthalmic management:
    - frequent lubricants

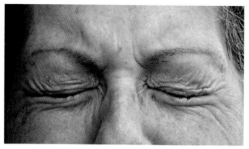

Fig. 7.27 Essential blepharospasm.

> taping the eyelids shut at night
> +/− lid surgery.
- Investigation of the cause of the nerve palsy.
- Specific treatment if possible.

EYELID SPASM (Fig. 7.27)

CAUSES

- Eyelid myokymia (eyelid twitching):
  > intermittent 'twitching' of one or both lids
  > a common, transient, benign condition that almost always resolves spontaneously.
- Essential blepharospasm (bilateral eyelid spasm):
  > repetitive forceful squeezing shut of both eyes.
- Hemifacial spasm (spasm of the eyelids and lower face on one side only):
  > repetitive forceful squeezing shut of one eye and contraction of the lower facial muscles on the same side.

MANAGEMENT

- Eyelid myokymia: reassure, await resolution.
- Essential blepharospasm or hemifacial spasm:
  > refer non-urgently to a neuro-ophthalmologist or neurologist
  > exclude an underlying eye disorder (e.g. severe dry eye)
  > 3-monthly botulinum toxin injections might alleviate the patient's symptoms.

WATERY, ITCHY OR GRITTY EYES

CHAPTER CONTENTS

OVERVIEW

These are probably the most common eye complaints and, in general, are the least serious (although often the most exasperating for both patient and practitioner!).

The most common cause of watery eye (epiphora) in young children is congenital nasolacrimal duct obstruction. This often resolves with age but might require probing under general anaesthetic as a curative procedure.

Itchy eyes are most commonly due to allergic conjunctivitis; gritty eyes are usually the result of dry eye or chronic mild eyelid inflammation (blepharitis). Foreign body sensation (the feeling that there is 'something in the eye') might be due to a corneal foreign body, early corneal ulcer, loose or inturned eyelashes, blepharitis, dry eye or a foreign body under the upper eyelid *(always evert ('flip') the upper eyelid in cases of unexplained foreign body sensation)*.

Watery, itchy or gritty eyes *Critical points*

- **Any patient with unexplained foreign body sensation requires ophthalmic referral** (urgently if there is also blurred vision, pain or photophobia).

- **A baby with watery eye(s)** probably has harmless nasolacrimal duct obstruction. However, **if photophobia, corneal clouding or corneal enlargement** are present the child should be suspected of having **congenital glaucoma** and be referred urgently.

WATERY EYE (EPIPHORA)

An eye can 'water' (overflow with tears, called epiphora) if:
- it is sore or irritated (reflex increase in tear production)
- the lacrimal drainage system is blocked (decrease in tear drainage).

The drainage system can become blocked at any level (see Fig. 2.6):
- Upper and lower lacrimal punctae (tear drainage 'holes' in the nasal part of the lid margins): these can close off in old age or be in the

wrong position to drain tears (e.g. if the lower lid is turned out in ectropion).
- Upper and lower lacrimal canaliculae (horizontal drainage tubes within the nasal part of the eyelids): these can be blocked by infection, trauma (eyelid lacerations) or age changes.
- The lacrimal sac in the bony outer wall of the nose and the vertical nasolacrimal duct, which connects the sac to the nose: this can be:
  - only partly canalised in babies (congenital nasolacrimal duct obstruction)
  - closed off in old age (age-related nasolacrimal duct obstruction).
- In nasolacrimal duct obstruction in children or adults, the lacrimal sac can:
  - become distended with trapped tears and mucus (mucocoele)
  - become infected (dacryocystitis).

WATERY EYE IN CHILDREN

The most common cause of this is congenital, idiopathic nasolacrimal duct blockage. Parents complain that their baby's eye(s) are always running or have a chronic sticky discharge.
Caution: **the following babies with 'watery eyes' require urgent referral**:
- **neonates with eye discharge**: to exclude ophthalmia neonatorum (see p. 105).
- **a baby with photophobia** (the child avoids bright lights), **corneal clouding** or **corneal enlargement** in addition to watering: to exclude congenital glaucoma.

Congenital nasolacrimal duct obstruction

- The nasolacrimal duct(s) fail to canalise before birth.

SIGNS

- Baby with watery, sticky or scant mucous discharge from one or both eyes.
- Otherwise normal eye(s) – not red or inflamed; the corneas are clear.
- Sometimes pressure over the lacrimal sac causes reflux of watery or mucous fluid through the lacrimal punctae in the eyelid margins.

MANAGEMENT

- If eyes otherwise normal: routine referral to ophthalmologist.
- Almost all cases will resolve spontaneously with time.
- If persisting at 12–18 months of age, nasolacrimal duct probing under a general anaesthetic is usually curative.

WATERY EYE IN ADULTS

Approach to an adult with watery eye(s)

- Is the eye sore or irritated? (possible reflex tearing due to eye disease, rather than obstructive epiphora)
- Are the eyes and eyelids normal?
  - corneal ulcer, corneal foreign body, blepharitis or ingrown eyelashes can cause reflex tearing.
- Are the lacrimal punctae normal, and in a normal position?
  - punctae can become narrowed or occluded with age (punctal stenosis)
  - the normal punctae are turned in to rest on the eyeball surface; if lower eyelid ectropion occurs (the lower lid is turned outwards) the lower punctum cannot drain tears as it is no longer in contact with the eye surface.

Age-related nasolacrimal duct obstruction

SYMPTOMS

- Watering (epiphora): tears can roll down the cheek; this can be embarrassing and annoying.

SIGNS

- The eye may appear constantly 'full of tears' or tears might run down the face.
- Otherwise normal eyes and eyelids.

MANAGEMENT

- Routine referral.

OPHTHALMIC MANAGEMENT

- Lacrimal canalicular probe/syringe: this is a diagnostic (not therapeutic) procedure in adults, to confirm whether obstruction is present.
- If duct obstruction confirmed and epiphora frequent, and the patient is keen for operation, dacryocystorhinostomy (DCR) can be performed. This bypasses the blocked duct by joining the lacrimal sac directly to the nasal cavity.

ITCHY EYES

This is most commonly due to allergic conjunctivitis in patients who also suffer from hayfever, asthma or eczema. Allergy can also develop to eye drops, contact lens solutions, make-up or other chemicals.

APPROACH TO A PATIENT WITH ITCHY EYES

ASK

- Is the problem present all year round, or is it seasonal?
- Is the patient an 'allergic' sort of person?
- Does the patient wear contact lenses?
- Does the patient use eye drops?
- Does the patient use make-up?

LOOK FOR

- Check the vision and corneas are normal.
- Evert (flip) the upper lid.
- Allergic conjunctivitis usually shows papillae (pink, cobblestone-like elevations under the upper lid).

ALLERGIC CONJUNCTIVITIS

See p. 95.

GRITTY EYES

Many patients with 'gritty' eyes have dry eyes or blepharitis.

DRY EYES

- This is common in elderly patients, and in younger patients with rheumatoid arthritis or other autoimmune diseases.
- It is commonly mild and irritating but, if severe, can threaten the sight if corneal ulceration occurs.

SYMPTOMS

- Dry/gritty/foreign body sensation.

SIGNS

- Eyes usually 'white' but might be red if severe.
- Usually no abnormality visible without a slit lamp.
- Slit lamp examination with fluorescein and blue light:
  - superficial punctate keratitis (many small yellow dots on the cornea) if moderate or severe.

MANAGEMENT

- If dry eyes *and mouth, and/or arthritis,* Sjögren's syndrome is likely:
  - refer to rheumatologist for assessment (this is a systemic disease that can cause other serious problems).
- Try common 'artificial tears' eye drops, every 2 hours initially, plus lubricating ointment at night.
- If no relief, routine ophthalmic referral.

BLEPHARITIS

- This is chronic irritation of the eyelid margins due to obstruction of the meibomian (lipid) glands and – sometimes – chronic colonisation of the lid margins by bacteria (Fig. 8.1).
- It might be an isolated finding or associated with a general disorder of the facial skin, such as acne rosacea.
- Blepharitis can cause complications such as marginal keratitis (see p. 98).

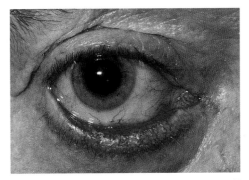

Fig. 8.1 Blepharitis: eyelid margin redness, thickening and scaling (lower lid ectropion is also present).

SYMPTOMS

● Chronic dry/gritty eyes, or foreign body sensation.

SIGNS

Magnification or slit lamp are helpful:
● Thickened lid margins.
● Lid telangiectasia (tortuous, fine, lid margin blood vessels).
● Blocking of meibomian gland orifices (these appear as a row of small white or yellow plugs on the lid margin).
● Scales on the eyelashes; loss of lashes can occur if severe.
● Facial skin changes of acne rosacea may be present, e.g. telangiectatic thickened red skin.

MANAGEMENT

● Twice a day lid hygiene (to help unblock the lipid glands and decrease the bacterial load):
  ▷ warm compress (e.g. warm damp face flannel) 5 minutes to the closed eyelids
  ▷ scrub the lid margins gently with a cotton bud dipped in diluted 'baby shampoo' (then rinse with water).
● Frequent artificial tears (every 2 hours if severe) can help if there is coexisting dry eye (which is common).
● If these measures do not help: routine ophthalmic referral.

FOREIGN BODY SENSATION

Foreign body sensation (the feeling that 'something is in the eye') can be the result of:

- Inturned eyelash(es).
- A foreign body:
  - under the top eyelid
  - between the lower eyelid and the eyeball
  - on the conjunctiva
  - on the cornea.
- Dry eye(s).
- Blepharitis.
- A small corneal abrasion or ulcer, e.g. marginal keratitis or recurrent erosion.

APPROACH TO A PATIENT WITH FOREIGN BODY SENSATION

ASK

- Did something blow or fly into the eye?
- Does the patient wear contact lenses? (could be an abrasion or ulcer)
- Has the patient had previous eye surgery? (could be a broken suture)

LOOK FOR

- Is the vision normal?
- Is the eye red?
- Look at the eyelids – are there inturned lashes?
- Look at the cornea for ulcer or foreign body. Then look again with fluorescein drops and a blue light.
- Look at the conjunctiva, ask the patient to look up, down, left and right – is there a foreign body?
- Pull the lower eyelid away from the eyeball and look for a foreign body on its inner surface.
- Evert (flip) the upper eyelid if you can't see any abnormality of the conjunctiva or cornea – an undetected foreign body might be trapped under the upper lid (see Fig. 2.12, p. 28, for the technique).

OTHER EYE SYMPTOMS

OVERVIEW

A patient might complain of eye symptoms other than those covered in the previous chapters. A frequent complaint from a middle-aged or elderly patient is of the sudden onset of 'floating spots' and/or 'flashing lights' in one eye: this has a greater than 90% chance of being a benign age-related change in the vitreous jelly, but it might herald a serious retinal tear or detachment. All these patients require urgent ophthalmic referral for a thorough retinal examination.

A patient can have normal central vision (visual acuity) but reduced peripheral vision (visual field loss), e.g. patients with pituitary tumours can present with complaints of blurred vision (due to loss of the temporal visual field in each eye) yet have 'normal' acuity on reading the letter chart. Visual field loss always signifies serious eye, optic nerve or brain disease. The various patterns of visual field loss are discussed below.

The symptoms and signs of temporal arteritis are included in this chapter because it is crucial that all practitioners can recognise the symptoms of this uncommon but potentially bilaterally blinding disease.

Other eye symptoms *Critical points*

- **New-onset 'flashes' and/or 'floaters' in one eye are a retinal detachment until proven otherwise – refer urgently.**

- **Not all flashing lights and headache is migraine –** occasionally, occipital tumours and vertebrobasilar transient ischaemic attacks can also cause flashes.

- **Every patient with blurred vision or headaches requires confrontation visual field testing.** This might be the only way to detect a brain tumour (e.g. pituitary tumour causing bitemporal hemianopia).

- **Visual field loss always requires ophthalmic assessment** (urgently if of sudden onset or if visual pathway disease is suspected) – it could be due to disease in the retina, optic nerve(s), or brain. *Continues*

Other eye symptoms *Critical points*—cont'd

- **Sudden-onset visual distortion (metamorphopsia)** is likely to be due to acute macular disease – refer urgently.

- **Temporal arteritis should be considered in every patient aged over 50 with one or more of:**
  - transient or persisting vision loss or double vision
  - new headaches, scalp tenderness on hair brushing, jaw muscle ache on chewing food, ear or neck pain, weight loss, fatigue, muscle aches
  - temporal arteries that are tender to palpation and/or not pulsatile
  - if suspicious: urgent referral.

FLOATING SPOTS

POSSIBLE CAUSES

- New floaters of sudden onset:
  - retinal tear or detachment
  - vitreous haemorrhage (e.g. bleeding from proliferative diabetic retinopathy)
  - age change in the vitreous jelly ('posterior vitreous detachment') – a harmless change if not associated with retinal tear.
- Long-standing floaters:
  - 'physiological' floaters (small clear floaters that most people notice if they look at a white wall or a blue sky).

APPROACH TO A PATIENT COMPLAINING OF FLOATING SPOTS IN THE VISION

ASK

- Are there flashes and/or field loss? (suspect retinal tear or detachment)
- Is the patient diabetic? (possible vitreous haemorrhage)
- Is the patient 'short-sighted' (myopic) or has he or she had previous cataract extraction? (increased risk of retinal tear or detachment)

LOOK FOR

- Is there a visual field defect to confrontation testing? (retinal detachment)
- Is there an afferent pupil defect? (retinal detachment)
- Is the red reflex normal and is there a clear view of the optic disc? (if not, vitreous haemorrhage or advanced retinal detachment could be present).
- 'Tobacco dust' (Fig. 9.1) might be visible on slit lamp examination if a retinal tear or detachment is present. These tiny brown particles of pigment can be seen in the vitreous behind the lens with the slit lamp after dilating drops have been used (this anterior part of the vitreous can be viewed directly with the slit lamp without having to use a hand-held lens).
- Does the retina look normal?
- *Note*: it is impossible to exclude retinal detachment with a direct ophthalmoscope because its field of view is too small.

'PHYSIOLOGICAL' FLOATERS

- Long-standing small floaters that most of us can see superimposed on a white wall or blue sky, or when reading.
- These are slight condensations in the normal vitreous jelly.

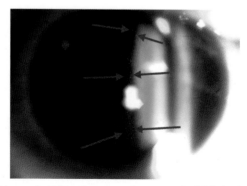

Fig. 9.1 'Tobacco dust' (tiny brown specks – arrows) visible in the anterior vitreous just behind the lens on slit lamp examination in a patient with a retinal tear.

POSTERIOR VITREOUS DETACHMENT (PVD)

- This is an age-related change in the vitreous jelly in which it breaks down into solid and liquid parts – the solid jelly peels off and separates from the retina.
- It causes new-onset floaters (often described as a black 'spider web' or 'net curtain') and often flashes of light ('like a camera flash out of the corner of my vision').

SIGNS

- Normal vision, no visual field defect to confrontation, no relative afferent pupil defect (RAPD).
- It is very difficult to see a posterior vitreous detachment without a dilated slit lamp retinal lens examination.

MANAGEMENT

- **Urgent referral to ophthalmologist** to exclude a retinal tear or detachment.
- Once serious retinal pathology has been excluded the patient can be reassured – no treatment is needed for the posterior vitreous detachment itself.

RETINAL TEAR

- A small percentage of posterior vitreous detachments create a retinal tear.

SYMPTOMS

- Identical to posterior vitreous detachment, i.e. flashes and floaters.
- Floaters might be large and black or red if the tear has caused vitreous haemorrhage.

MANAGEMENT

- **Urgent ophthalmic referral.**
- If a tear is found, it is 'welded shut' with laser burns to prevent a retinal detachment developing.

RETINAL DETACHMENT

See p. 51.

VITREOUS HAEMORRHAGE

See p. 53.

FLASHING LIGHTS

POSSIBLE CAUSES

- Retina:
  - retinal tear (see above)
  - retinal detachment (see p. 51)
  - age change in the vitreous jelly (posterior vitreous detachment; see above).
- Brain:
  - migraine headache (see p. 45)
  - 'acephalgic' migraine (migraine with the visual prodrome but no headache)
  - (rarely) posterior circulation (occipital lobe) transient ischaemic attacks
  - (rarely) occipital lobe tumour or vascular malformation.

APPROACH TO A PATIENT COMPLAINING OF FLASHING LIGHTS IN THE VISION

ASK

- The patient to describe the visual symptoms:
  - flashing/flickering white lights in one eye ('like lightning flashes'): likely vitrcoretinal cause
  - transient patch of blurred vision reported as being in one or two eyes with 'zig-zag' lines, 'sparkling' lights or coloured lights: more likely brain cause.
- Is there a history of headaches consistent with true migraine and/or a family history of migraine?

LOOK FOR

- Is there a visual field defect to confrontation testing?
  - if present in one eye: likely retinal detachment
  - if homonymous field loss present (the same side of both visual fields): possible occipital tumour or stroke.
- Is there an afferent pupil defect? (retinal detachment).
- Red reflex and ophthalmoscopy.
- Check blood pressure.
- Any neurological signs?

VISUAL FIELD LOSS

POSSIBLE CAUSES

- Retina:
  - retinal detachment (see p. 51)
  - retinal vascular occlusion (see p. 47)
  - other disease.
- Optic nerve:
  - advanced chronic glaucoma (see p. 72)
  - optic nerve disease of any other cause.
- Brain:
  - optic chiasm, optic radiation or occipital lobe disease.

APPROACH TO A PATIENT WITH VISUAL FIELD LOSS

ASK

- Is the loss in one or both eyes?
  - one eye: likely retinal or optic nerve disease
  - both eyes: likely brain disease.
- What part of the visual field is affected in each eye? (right, left, upper, lower, or centre?)
- How was the visual field loss noticed?
  - on accidentally covering the other eye?
  - as a slowly-increasing 'shadow' or 'curtain' in one eye? (likely retinal detachment).
- Are there flashes and floaters in one eye? (likely retinal detachment).
- Are there flashes simultaneously in both eyes? (possible occipital brain disease).
- Does the patient have any neurological symptoms?

LOOK FOR

- Is the vision decreased on testing?
- Is there a visual field defect to confrontation testing?
  - in one or both eyes?
  - what is the pattern of the field defect?
- Is there an afferent pupil defect? (retinal detachment or optic nerve disease)
- Is the red reflex normal and is there a clear view of the optic disc?
  - *Note*: retinal detachment cannot be excluded with a direct ophthalmoscope because its field of view is too small.

- Does the patient have high blood pressure?
- Are there any neurological signs?

PATTERNS OF VISUAL FIELD LOSS

See Fig. 2.7, p. 18 and Fig. 9.2.

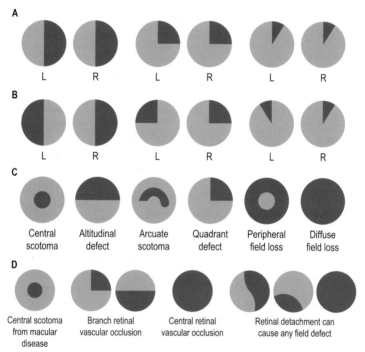

Fig. 9.2 The different patterns of visual field loss. **A**, Field defects from retrochiasmal disease: right homonymous hemianopic field defects from left side retrochiasmal disease; **B**, field defects from optic chiasm disease: bitemporal hemianopic field defects from optic chiasm disease (usually compression by a pituitary tumour); **C**, field defects from optic nerve disease: one or both eyes may be affected (if both, there are often different defects in each eye); optic nerve disease of any type can cause any of these defects; **D**, field defects from retinal disease.

General rules

- Visual field loss *stopping at the horizontal midline* is often caused by *retinal or optic nerve disease*, e.g. branch retinal vascular occlusions, glaucoma, optic neuropathies of any cause.

- Visual field loss *stopping at the vertical midline* is often caused by disease of the visual pathways in the *brain*.

- However, note:
  - optic nerve disease of almost *any* kind can cause almost *any* type of visual field defect
  - compression of the optic nerve(s) by a brain tumour can cause *any* pattern of visual field loss, in *one or both* eyes
  - no type of visual field defect is 'diagnostic' for a particular type of optic nerve disease.

- Disease anterior to the chiasm on one side (retina or optic nerve disease) causes field loss of any pattern in one eye only (although field loss may be bilateral if both optic nerves are affected).

- Disease in the chiasm (e.g. chiasm compression due to a pituitary tumour) often causes a partial or complete bitemporal hemianopia (loss of the temporal (outer) side of both visual fields).

- Disease posterior to the chiasm on one side (retrochiasmal brain disease) often causes a homonymous hemianopia (loss of the same side of both visual fields) on the side opposite the brain lesion, i.e. a right occipital stroke will cause a left homonymous hemianopia (loss of the left hemifield of the left eye, and the left hemifield of the right eye).

DISTORTED VISION

This is usually due to macular (central retinal) disease. Patients might report that lines of book print 'run into each other' or that straight lines, such as doorframes, appear to 'curve'.

POSSIBLE CAUSES

IN ELDERLY PATIENTS

- Gradual onset, slow progression:
  - dry age-related macular degeneration (ARMD; see p. 67): no treatment possible
  - epiretinal membrane (age-related scar tissue on the surface of the retina) or age-related macular hole: surgical treatment might help.
- Sudden onset, rapid progression: wet age-related macular degeneration (see p. 57): possible laser treatment.

IN YOUNGER PATIENTS

- Diabetic maculopathy (see p. 68).
- Central serous retinopathy.

APPROACH TO A PATIENT WITH DISTORTED VISION

- Does the patient report distortion of the lines on an Amsler grid (see Fig. 2.18, p. 34) or a sheet of ruled paper?
- Macular disease does *not* usually cause a relative afferent pupil defect.
- On ophthalmoscopy after dilating eye drops:
  - haemorrhages, exudates or swelling might be visible at the macula
  - *note*: the direct ophthalmoscope is *not* the ideal instrument for macular examination.

PAIN AROUND THE EYE

Not all pain in or around the eye is from the eye. If the eye is not red and has normal vision – and if there is no relative afferent pupil defect, proptosis or double vision – the eye is unlikely to be the source of the pain.

POSSIBLE DIAGNOSES

- Eye disease, e.g. iritis, acute glaucoma, acute optic neuritis.
- Orbit disease, e.g. orbital inflammation or tumour.
- Referred pain:
  - trigeminal nerve:
    - irritation or compression of the nerve by tumour or inflammation
    - idiopathic trigeminal neuralgia
  - other intracranial disease, e.g. aneurysm, inflammation
  - nasal sinus disease
  - idiopathic headache syndromes, e.g. cluster headache.

APPROACH TO A PATIENT WITH PAIN AROUND THE EYE

ASK

- Does the patient have blurred vision?
- Does the patient have double vision?
- Is the pain in the eye or around it?
- What is the nature of the pain? ('shooting' or 'electric' pains suggest neuralgia – either primary or secondary).
- Does the patient have any other neurological or sinus symptoms?

LOOK FOR

- Visual acuity/signs of eye disease (e.g. redness, afferent pupil defect).
- Signs of orbit disease (e.g. proptosis, limitation of eye movement).
- Signs of intracranial disease:
  - test corneal and facial sensation and cranial nerves; if sensation is decreased there is a significant chance an intracranial tumour is present.
- Signs of nasal sinus disease.

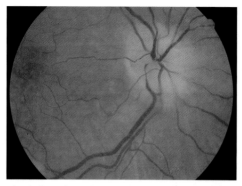

Fig. 9.3 Anterior ischaemic optic neuropathy (AION) due to temporal arteritis.

SYMPTOMS OF TEMPORAL ARTERITIS

Patients often complain of headache. A few of these patients will have temporal arteritis (also called 'giant cell' arteritis), an uncommon but serious vasculitic disease that **occurs only in adults over the age of 50.** This condition frequently causes **permanent blindness of one or both eyes** if not identified and treated promptly.

Ideally, temporal arteritis is diagnosed *before* visual loss occurs, and adequate oral steroid treatment can usually *prevent* visual loss (once visual loss has occurred, it is usually irreversible). It is important that all practitioners are aware of this disease and of the cardinal signs and symptoms that distinguish it from other causes of headache.

COMPLICATIONS

Temporal arteritis can cause:
- Transient visual loss (amaurosis fugax).
- Persisting visual loss, most commonly by causing anterior ischaemic optic neuropathy (infarction of the optic nerve head; Fig. 9.3) and less commonly because it causes central or branch retinal artery occlusion.
- Transient double vision.
- Persisting double vision (by causing an ischaemic third, fourth or sixth nerve palsy, or orbital ischaemia).
- Stroke, heart attack or bowel infarction.

SYMPTOMS

One or more of:
- A *new* type of headache (that the patient hasn't had previously).
- Scalp tenderness on hair brushing.
- Jaw muscle ache on chewing food.
- Ear or neck pain.
- Weight loss, fatigue, muscle aches.
- Symptoms of ophthalmic or systemic complications.

SIGNS

- The temporal arteries (at the sides of the forehead) might be tender and/or not pulsatile on palpation.
- Signs of the above complications.

MANAGEMENT

- **Urgent ophthalmic referral if visual symptoms are present.**
- **If no visual symptoms, urgent rheumatological referral.**

OPHTHALMIC MANAGEMENT

- Urgent assessment and blood test for erythrocyte sedimentation rate (ESR) and C-reactive protein (CRP) (these are usually markedly elevated).
- Immediate high-dose oral steroid treatment to protect the vision (this continues on a tapering dose for at least 1 year).
- Temporal artery biopsy within a few days, for histological confirmation of the diagnosis.

CHAPTER 10

WHO NEEDS SCREENING FOR EYE DISEASE?

CHAPTER CONTENTS

OVERVIEW

Many people in the community require regular eye examinations, even if their vision is completely normal. This could be because:

- The eye disease they are at risk of can significantly damage peripheral vision before they become aware of it (e.g. glaucoma).
- The disease is best and most safely treated if caught at an early (presymptomatic) stage (e.g. diabetic retinopathy).
- The patients at risk are preverbal children who are unable to communicate their decrease in vision to those around them.

In addition, all children require at least a red reflex examination at birth and a preschool or early school vision check. Glaucoma experts also recommend that all adults over age 40 have regular glaucoma checks.

Who needs screening for eye disease? **Critical points**

- **All patients with diabetes require a careful retinal examination at diagnosis, and then yearly for the rest of their lives.** A direct ophthalmoscope examination is not adequate for screening as it can miss early or moderate diabetic maculopathy.

- **All adults over age 40 should have a glaucoma screening test (intraocular pressure and optic disc examination) by their optometrist every 2 years for the rest of their lives.** Patients who have close relatives with glaucoma should obtain ophthalmic advice regarding the age at which screening should begin.

- Certain other patients benefit from routine eye screening: see below.

CHILDREN

ALL CHILDREN

Routine eye checks for all children:

- Red reflex at birth (by the examining paediatrician or hospital doctor):
  - to check for congenital cataracts or other major congenital eye problems
  - if cataracts are identified and operated on in the first few weeks of life, the child might avoid severe bilateral amblyopic visual loss.
- Preschool or early school vision check, to detect:
  - squint: if not detected and treated early, this can cause amblyopia
  - refractive error: without the correct glasses, the child could find schoolwork difficult and/or develop amblyopia.

PREMATURE INFANTS

- Selected premature babies will have screening by an ophthalmologist in hospital for retinopathy of prematurity (ROP), which can be treated with laser if detected early.
- The lower the gestational age and the lower the birth weight, the greater the risk.

MATERNAL INFECTIONS DURING PREGNANCY

- Maternal infections such as rubella, cytomegalovirus (CMV), toxoplasmosis and syphilis during pregnancy can have major effects on the baby's developing visual system.
- The babies of mothers who are symptomatic for these infections, or who are positive on routine testing, require ophthalmic examination soon after birth to detect any congenital eye abnormalities, which might be treatable. For example, congenital rubella often causes infantile cataracts and, if these are removed early in life, vision can be saved.

FAMILY HISTORY OF CHILDHOOD EYE DISEASE

- Some eye diseases such as high refractive error, congenital cataracts, retinoblastoma and idiopathic strabismus 'run' strongly in families.
- For this reason, the children of a parent with a history of a congenital or childhood eye disease should have the appropriate screening examinations.

CHILDREN WITH A HEAD TILT

- Congenital or acquired fourth nerve palsy is a common cause of head tilt in childhood.
- If this is not detected early, the tilt might become long standing and even cause secondary permanent bony changes in the neck and face.
- Hence any child with a persistent head tilt or turn requires an ophthalmic examination to exclude a fourth nerve palsy.

ANY CHILD WITH ARTHRITIS

- Juvenile idiopathic arthritis (previously called juvenile rheumatoid arthritis) is often associated with iritis.
- Unlike adult iritis, this form of iritis in children does not cause the eye(s) to become red and young children are unreliable in reporting visual loss. Thus this form of iritis can be detected only by routine screening examinations by an ophthalmologist.

DOWN SYNDROME

- Children with Down syndrome have an increased risk of many eye diseases, including cataract, squint, refractive error and keratoconus. The child can benefit greatly if these are treated early in life.
- Adults with Down syndrome might develop cataract much earlier than other adults.

NEUROFIBROMATOSIS

- This condition has a greatly increased risk of optic nerve and orbital tumours and affected children require ophthalmic screening.
- Children who have a parent with neurofibromatosis also require screening, as the disease has autosomal dominant inheritance.

HIV

- As with adults, children with HIV require screening for cytomegalovirus (CMV) retinopathy once severe immunodeficiency is reached.

MEDICATIONS

Ophthalmic examination is required before beginning (or soon after starting) these drugs, and at regular intervals during treatment:

- Tuberculosis treatment – ethambutol, isoniazid: often cause a toxic optic neuropathy.
- Hydroxychloroquine (e.g. for arthritis or systemic lupus erythematosus): this can cause a toxic maculopathy if used in moderate or high doses for a prolonged period.
- Vigabatrin (for epilepsy): can cause a toxic retinopathy, with initial loss of peripheral vision.
- Other drugs might also require eye screening: check the prescribing information.

CHILDREN WITH DEVELOPMENTAL DELAY OR EDUCATIONAL PROBLEMS

- Squint and refractive error are often unfairly blamed for children's learning disabilities and poor performance at school.
- However children with developmental problems need at least one eye test, to ensure that poor vision is not a contributing factor.

ADULTS

ALL ADULTS

- Chronic glaucoma is common in middle-aged and elderly adults. It is asymptomatic until advanced visual field loss has occurred.
- It has been recommended that **all adults over the age of 40 have a glaucoma screening check every 2 years for the rest of their lives by their optometrist.**
- An intraocular pressure measurement and optic disc examination should be a routine part of every optometrist's 'glasses check' examination; it is not necessary to perform formal visual field testing if the pressure and discs are normal.
- Patients with a family history of chronic glaucoma should be especially strongly encouraged to have regular screening; if their relatives were diagnosed at a young age they might need to begin screening much younger than 40 (ask ophthalmic advice).

ALL PATIENTS WITH DIABETES

Diabetes can cause decreased vision in two main ways:

- *Diabetic maculopathy* (see p. 68): a common cause of gradual visual loss in diabetics:
  - swelling of the macula (the central retinal area) occurs due to leakage of fluid from retinal blood vessels
  - this is best treated with laser when detected at an early stage, when vision might be normal or only slightly decreased, in an effort to prevent severe visual loss from chronic macular changes.
- *Proliferative diabetic retinopathy* (see p. 176): abnormal new retinal vessels grow from the retina into the vitreous:
  - this can cause vitreous haemorrhage (sudden onset of floaters +/– visual loss) or traction retinal detachment (gradual or sudden visual loss)
  - it is vital that proliferative diabetic retinopathy is detected and treated with laser at an early stage (*before* symptoms due to vitreous haemorrhage or retinal detachment occur) if visual loss is to be prevented.

  All diabetics should have a retinal screening examination at diagnosis, and then on a regular basis for life. Screening is usually annual or more frequent if severe disease is present.

ONE-EYED PATIENTS

One-eyed patients (or patients with only one 'good' eye) should have a yearly or second-yearly eye check by their optometrist to detect treatable disease (e.g. glaucoma) in the only seeing eye.

PATIENTS WITH HIV

Patients with HIV who have severe immunodeficiency require regular screening for cytomegalovirus (CMV) retinopathy.

MEDICATIONS

- Ethambutol or isoniazid (for tuberculosis treatment): these often cause toxic optic neuropathy.
- Hydroxychloroquine (for rheumatoid arthritis or systemic lupus erythematosus): can cause toxic maculopathy.
- Tamoxifen (for breast cancer): can cause a toxic maculopathy.
- Vigabatrin (for epilepsy): can cause a toxic retinopathy – loss of peripheral vision first (ophthalmic screening involves serial examination and visual field testing).
- Other drugs can also cause ocular toxicity and require screening: check the prescribing information.

Your local pharmaceutical guide will outline any local recommendations for screening adults on these medications. Particular care must be taken with patients with communication difficulties, who might be unable to explain that their vision is worsening.

BASIC EYE PROCEDURES

CHAPTER CONTENTS

DOUBLE EYE PATCH APPLICATION

INDICATIONS

- After removal of a corneal foreign body.
- Non-infected corneal abrasion.
- For 'weld flash' burn.

TECHNIQUE

- Have two eye patches and five 15-cm pieces of adhesive tape cut and ready.
- Put a small amount of antibiotic ointment onto the eye (pull down lower lid, ask the patient to look up and place ointment in the groove between the inside of the lid and the eye).
- Ask the patient to close both eyes.
- Fold the first patch over on itself lengthways and place it over the eye so the straight side fits in the top of the eye socket and the curved side is at the bottom (Fig. 11.1, top left).
- Place the second patch (unfolded) vertically over the first (Fig. 11.1, top right).
- Stick the first piece of tape firmly to the forehead, then to the pad, then to the cheek.
- Repeat for the other pieces of tape – the patch should be completely covered and surrounded with tape (Fig. 11.1, bottom left).
- **The patch should be tight enough to hold the eyelids *closed* underneath.** The patient should not be able to open the eye when the pad is complete:
  - a loose eye patch will do more harm than good (it could cause a corneal abrasion when the eye opens under it).
- **Review and remove the patch within 24 hours** – never leave a patch on for longer than a day.
- If the abrasion or epithelial defect is healing but still present, re-apply a fresh patch again after re-examination.

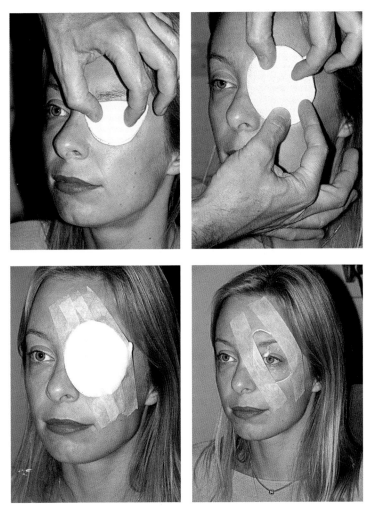

Fig. 11.1 Applying a double eye patch (top left, top right, bottom left). Bottom right: an eye shield (use instead of a patch in suspected penetrating eye injury).

CORNEAL FOREIGN BODY REMOVAL

Do not attempt removal yourself but instead refer urgently to an eye emergency department if:

- You are concerned the foreign body could be **full-thickness** through the cornea (e.g. a wood or metal splinter).
- There are signs of **infection.**
- The foreign body is **central** in the cornea (i.e. the size of the scar from removal will be visually important) or deep.

TECHNIQUE FOR FOREIGN BODY REMOVAL

- Do this yourself only if there are *no* signs of infection and *no* suspicion of penetrating eye injury.
- It is ideal to remove foreign bodies while viewing through a slit lamp. However, if this is not available it can often be performed with other magnification or even macroscopically (if you have good near vision).
- Examine the eyes and test visual acuity.
- If you do not have access to a slit lamp, lie the patient down with the head well supported.
- Put several drops of local anaesthetic (e.g. Benoxinate) on the cornea, each a minute apart (warn the patient this will sting initially).
- Try to gently wipe the foreign body off with a sterile cotton bud first – this often works.
- If this does not work, try to remove the foreign body under good light with a short 25-G needle on a small syringe (to use as a handle).
- **Remember, it is always better to refer the patient for slit lamp removal than to cause corneal scarring or perforation by overzealous attempts at removal.**
- Antibiotic ointment and double eye patch (see above); review within 24 hours.
- Refer to an eye emergency department if the foreign body (or rust ring around it) cannot to be removed completely (going back and having another try tomorrow usually doesn't help).

EYE IRRIGATION

INDICATIONS

Chemical burn to the eye.

TECHNIQUE

- **Commence irrigation** (Fig. 11.2) **immediately**, *before examination.*
- Put several drops of local anaesthetic (e.g. Benoxinate) into the eyes to allow the patient to open them.
- Irrigate the eyes continuously with clean running fluid: normal saline (a drip bag on a pole) or running water (via a hose or even using a series of water jugs) for 30 minutes (unless extensive irrigation has already been performed).
- Put a kidney dish or bowl under the ear(s) to catch the run-off fluid.
- While irrigating, evert the upper and lower lids, irrigate under them and remove any particles of foreign matter with a cotton bud (this is particularly important if the chemical is a powder).
- Once the irrigation is complete, instil more local anaesthetic and examine the eyes carefully.
- We *do not* recommend:
  - testing the eye pH with paper strips
  - using any 'antidote' chemicals
  - using 'irrigating contact lenses'.

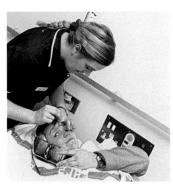

Fig. 11.2 Eye irrigation.

FURTHER READING

Kanski J J. Clinical ophthalmology, 5th edn. Oxford, Butterworth Heinemann, 2003. 748 pages.
An excellent comprehensive reference of ophthalmic diseases for optometrists; an ideal first text for medical students or hospital doctors wishing to pursue ophthalmology training.

Yanoff M, Duker J S. Ophthalmology, 2nd edn. St Louis, Mosby, 2004. 1552 pages.
A more advanced general reference text.

INDEX